GABRIEL'S ANGELS

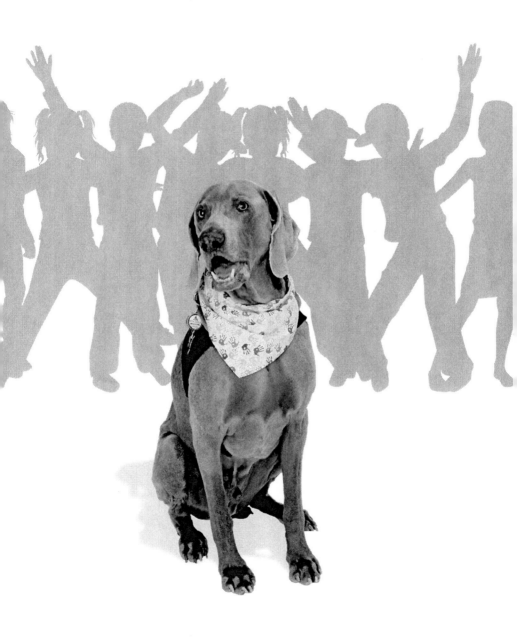

Stay Inspired !

Pam
5 /2011

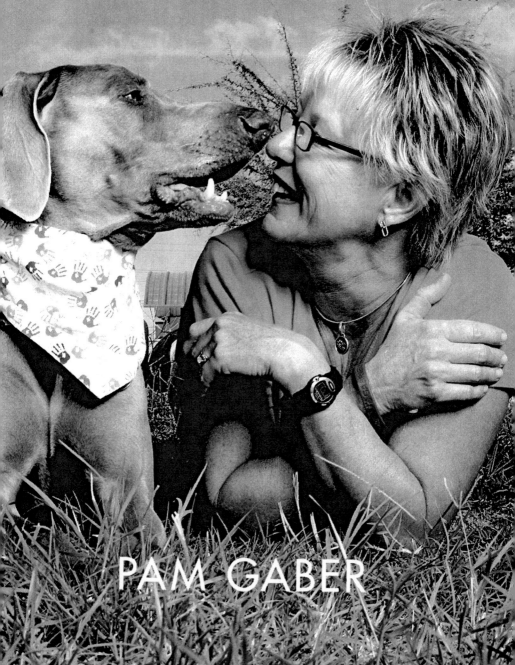

GABRIEL'S ANGELS

THE STORY OF THE DOG WHO INSPIRED A REVOLUTION

PAM GABER

Praise for GABRIEL'S ANGELS

Comments from agencies Gabriel's Angels serves

"The difference Gabriel's Angels has made to our children and our program is nothing short of phenomenal. The children have learned empathy, unconditional love and self-control as a result of their interactions with Gabriel'sAngels." — *Crisis Nursery, Phoenix*

"The children are able to verbalize the dogs' attributes and needs. They are able to cooperate and take turns with responsibilities."
— *Casa de los Ninos, Tucson*

"The kids play with new children when the therapy dog is here. They are kinder to one another and more open to new friendships."
— *La Mesita Child & Youth Center, Mesa*

"Students have less behavioral issues and emotional outbursts during visits." — *Madison Meadows School*

"Our Therapy Team creates an atmosphere for our students to get to know each other more quickly by experiencing the dogs' unconditional love during their visits. I witnessed documented criminal gang members give attention and gentle pats to the therapy dogs."
— *Pinnacle High School, Mesa*

"Gabriel's Angels provides a non-threatening venue to learn self-control and sensitivity." — *South Pointe Elementary School, Phoenix*

"This program has boosted the kids' self-esteem."
— *Rosenzweig Boys and Girls Club, Phoenix*

"A 10-year-old boy was displaying aggressive behaviors with other children. After three therapy visits, his aggressive behavior was controlled."
— *CAAFA, Apache Junction*

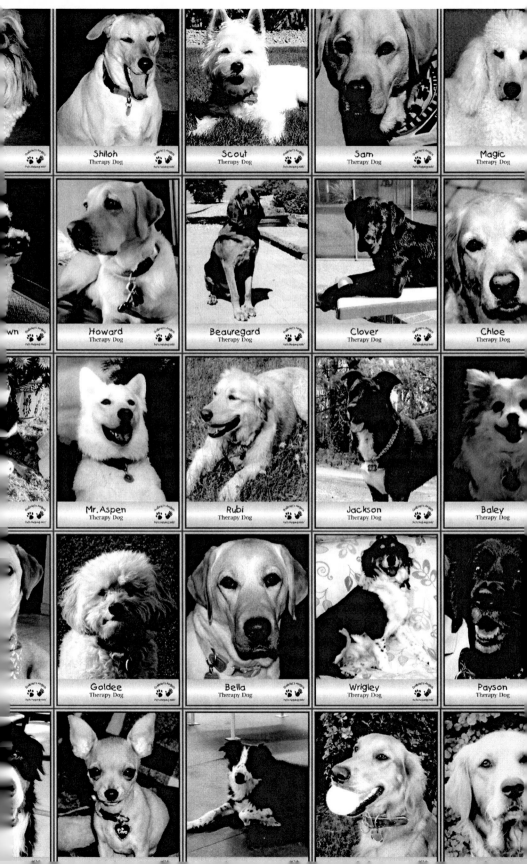

Shiloh
Therapy Dog

Scout
Therapy Dog

Sam
Therapy Dog

Magic
Therapy Dog

Howard
Therapy Dog

Beauregard
Therapy Dog

Clover
Therapy Dog

Chloe
Therapy Dog

Mr. Aspen
Therapy Dog

Rubi
Therapy Dog

Jackson
Therapy Dog

Baley
Therapy Dog

Goldee
Therapy Dog

Bella
Therapy Dog

Wrigley
Therapy Dog

Payson
Therapy Dog

Praise for GABRIEL'S ANGELS

Comments from children Gabriel's Angels has served

"I have a dog at home, and when she was young I would get really angry, and if I get really angry I take it out ... I take it out on my dog, but now I see I was really wrong. I don't want to hurt a dog again. They're too loveable. I just don't want to hurt them again."
— *Kyle, age 14*

"What I learned was you need to take care of them and pick up after them and give them a bath and take them for walks." — *Michael, age 8*

"Thank you for bringing Noah. My favorite part is when we petted him." — *Daniel, age 6*

"I love the dogs that play with us and that teach us that they are like us. They show me how to show empathy to humans and dogs and other living creatures." — *Lucinda, age 15*

"I get that you learn to respect human boundaries as well as dog boundaries. You learn to love. That is what I get out of [Gabriel's Angels visits]. — *Corey, age 14*

From when Gabriel was unable to visit due to chemotherapy: "I love him and miss him and I hope he has a good day. When I grow up, I'm going to buy him a house and a bone." — *Michael, age 5*

"Why I originally started abusing dogs was because of all my frustrations — it's like a scapegoat. I would use them to get what I wanted. After ... ever since doing years of experience with Jack and all the other Gabriel's Angels members, I finally get it and I won't do that again." — *Ryan, age 15*

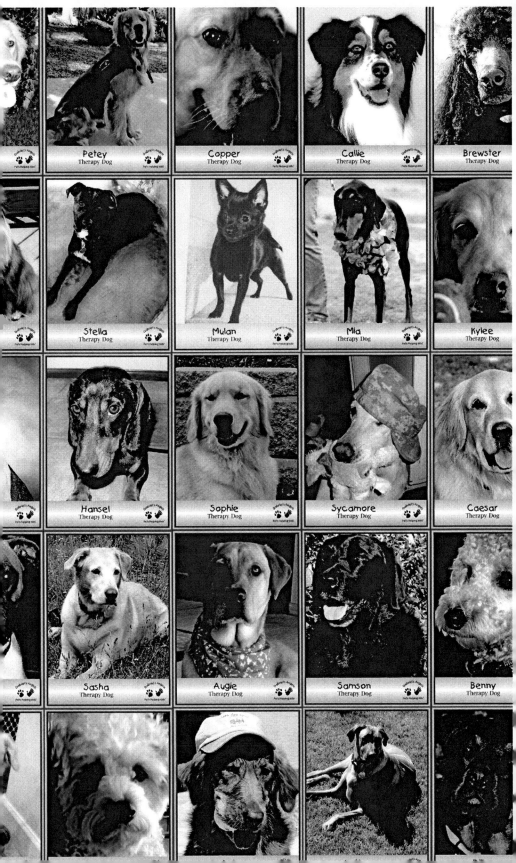

Praise for GABRIEL'S ANGELS

Quotes from sympathy cards received after Gabriel passed away

"Gabriel created a movement of hope for children."

"Gabriel is playing with all the kids in Heaven."

"I hope you see Gabriel in the smiling faces of the children you help every day."

"Gabriel has been preparing most of his life to be one of God's angels. It is impossible to measure his positive impact on Arizona's children and the generations that will follow."

"Because of Gabe, thousands of children know kindness and compassion."

"His life will touch generations to come."

"How inspiring, your life together and the love and joy you brought to all you touched. What a legacy you created together ... your angel, Gabriel, that you shared with everyone."

"Gabriel's gift of helping children will live on — very few are fortunate enough to have such a legacy."

"Pam, you and Gabriel symbolize what a gifted dog and committed person can do to bring healing to those in need."

"Pam, Gabriel was truly an angel to everyone whose lives he touched — we all miss him." *—Stephanie at FACES* (a facility Gabriel visited)

"Miss Pam — Thank you for sharing Gabriel with us here at the shelter. We will miss you, Gabriel, and will always have your memory in our hearts." *—Your Friends at Crisis Nursery*

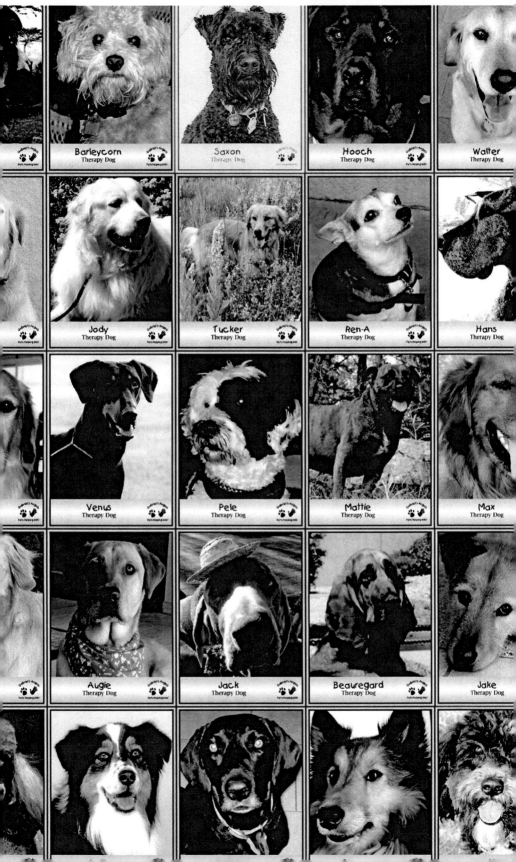

Barleycorn
Therapy Dog

Saxon
Therapy Dog

Hooch
Therapy Dog

Walter
Therapy Dog

Jody
Therapy Dog

Tucker
Therapy Dog

Ren-A
Therapy Dog

Hans
Therapy Dog

Venus
Therapy Dog

Pele
Therapy Dog

Mattie
Therapy Dog

Max
Therapy Dog

Augie
Therapy Dog

Jack
Therapy Dog

Beauregard
Therapy Dog

Jake
Therapy Dog

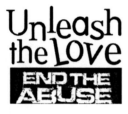

Gabriel's Angels, Inc.

1550 E. Maryland Avenue, Suite 1

Phoenix, Arizona 85014

GabrielsAngels.org

602.266.0875

ISBN 978-0-615-44590-8

LCNN 2011926167

This book is dedicated to the Gabriel's Angels volunteer therapy
teams who were inspired to follow in Gabriel's pawprints.
By giving of themselves and their dogs, they have impacted the lives
of more than 50,000 Arizona children since we opened in 2000.
I would be remiss if I did not also thank our amazing board of directors,
steering committee, and staff, who continue to inspire me every day.

Godspeed, Big Gray.

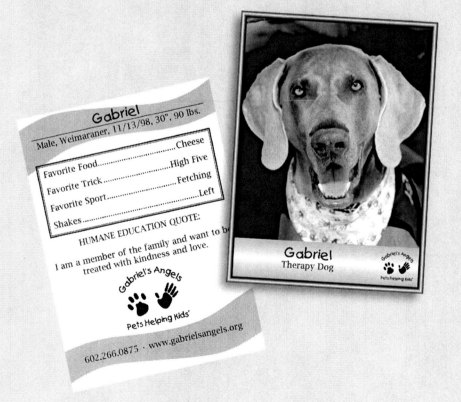

Gabriel
Male, Weimaraner, 11/13/98, 30", 90 lbs.

Favorite Food..Cheese
Favorite Trick..................................High Five
Favorite Sport....................................Fetching
Shakes...Left

HUMANE EDUCATION QUOTE:
I am a member of the family and want to be
treated with kindness and love.

Gabriel's Angels
Pets Helping Kids®

602.266.0875 · www.gabrielsangels.org

Gabriel
Therapy Dog

Gabriel's Angels
Pets Helping Kids®

Preface

I've always felt there were two kinds of writers — those who wrote effortlessly with great imagination and who made it their profession. The others were those who had something amazing or tragic happen in their lives and needed to tell their story. I am in the latter cateogry. I had something amazing happen to me, and while not a natural or professional writer, felt compelled to tell the story of the dog who inspired a revolution. "A revolution?" you may be asking. "How could a dog do that?"

Throughout the years, I've heard from many people, "You must write a book about Gabriel's Angels. It is an amazing story, Pam." Somehow, I could never get started — writer's block perhaps? Or maybe I didn't know how this amazing story would end. Quite frankly, I didn't document the events of the past eleven-and-a-half years, and the thought of trying to remember everything was overwhelming.

Upon the death of the dog who inspired this revolution, I felt the need to tell his story and credit him with all he accomplished and the many lives he touched. Suddenly I was inspired to write this book, both for him and for me. This is Gabriel's legacy tribute. His story will move you from laughter to tears. He lived a full, adventurous life, and he touched the lives of more than 10,000 abused, neglected, and at-risk children through his work as a therapy dog. I want to share him with you.

I also wrote this book for myself. I hoped it would be healing, as Gabriel's passing created a huge void in my life. We realize, when a puppy enters our life, that we will have ten, twelve, or even fifteen years of unconditional love. We also know that woman's best friend does not live forever. Yet somehow we live in denial, going about life ignoring their graying muzzles and achy joints. Is it because dogs give so unconditionally that their hearts wear out way too soon?

GABRIEL'S ANGELS

I learned much from my big gray dog, and I hope you will, too. Writing this book has been a labor of love and involved many special people. You will hear from Gabriel's veterinarian who did his first puppy exam and ultimately ended his suffering. Supporters from our board of directors and the community express their appreciation for Gabriel's work. One young man remembers, many years later, how a gentle gray dog impacted his life. You will also read the story of my sweet mom who was battling sudden late-stage cancer and could not be told of Gabriel's passing because she was too weak.

I began this book-writing journey two months after Gabriel passed away. It has been both a joy and a burden. I wish to express my gratitude to all who helped me along the way.

To my husband, Mike, who supported my efforts and is my biggest cheerleader. His heart was broken when we lost Gabriel, and still is. I don't know if he will ever get over it. Mike was the "fun" parent, in Gabriel's view. I was the disciplinarian but took Gabriel to visit the kids, which put me in a good light, too.

I am so appreciative of my last eight months working with my copywriter/editor, Laura Orsini, Owner and Creative Director of Write I Market I Design, to birth this book. I am grateful for her intense desire to make the book the best it could be. We spent hours recording interviews which were transcribed, organized, and returned to me so I could review the text. I disciplined myself to complete what I had promised to do — write the inspirational and true story of Gabriel's life. I felt his presence as I worked in my office every weekend to stay on schedule. I think he is proud of me.

My amazing designer extraordinaire, Bill Greaves, brought Gabe's book to life. He is an artistic genius who instinctively knew the best way to add the visual dimension of Gabriel's story. While I supplied the words, Bill created the masterful design that resulted in the finished product.

To everyone else who contributed to this book: Dr. Betsy, Cassie, Dr. Christina, Dr. Dean, Debbie, Diane, Ernest, Ilana, Jan, Linda, Marsha, Mary Jo, Lissa, Phil A., Phil F., Sage, Robert, and Dr. Wayne. Thank you for your time and desire to help me.

Another big thank you to all the nonprofit agencies that welcome our pet therapy teams; if not for them, we would not be here today.

And finally, thank you to our entire community for supporting our efforts over the past ten years. I look forward to growing together.

Welcome to the journey of a gentle gray dog named Gabriel who inspired a revolution. I am happy to have you along for the ride.

—*Pam*

Table of Contents

CHAPTER ONE

The Adoption

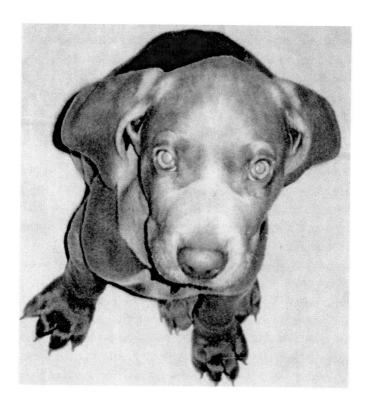

All I wanted was a puppy.

For my whole life, I'd just loved animals. I remember growing up, we had a big dog named Fluffy, and he heard all my tales of woe. He even told me I was right when my mom said I was wrong. Fluffy and I had a bond. He was a black and white party poodle, and I experienced such unconditional love from him. I remember the wagging of the tail when I came home, and as an adult, I missed all that. I had two cats who were beautiful companions, but there's something about a dog and the way dogs connect. I wanted one, but my busy, busy work schedule didn't allow it. Once I left Corporate America, though, I was ready. My husband had a schnauzer as a young boy, but I was the animal girl. He loved our cats, but I knew getting a dog would be good for Mike, too.

It was New Year's Day 1999 when Mike and I went "puppy-looking." What is puppy-looking? "We're going to adopt a puppy today," is what it turns out to mean.

Mike and I had been talking over the Christmas holiday, and I told him, "I want a puppy." But long hair was out. A little dog was out. I love big, boy dogs. I wanted a big lug of a dog that could hike and run with us. We decided to look at two breeds, Weimaraners and Vizslas.

We found a Weimaraner breeder and trekked off to Gilbert, Arizona, a suburb of Phoenix, and drove up to this little house. It was a smaller house — maybe a 1,500 square foot home. It turned out there were six puppies, two adult Weimaraners, several kids, and two adults living there. It was bedlam!

The two Weimaraner parents were very friendly — and I mean VERY friendly. The puppies were playing and running everywhere. I was in shock, because remember, I had cats, and cats don't do that. Cats are very calm. These dogs were hyper with a capital H. I was so out of my element at this point, yet we stayed.

January in Phoenix can be much warmer than other parts of the country, so I was wearing shorts because it was a nice day. We asked the owners to take the adults away so we could focus on the out-of-control puppies. They told us that out of a litter of twelve, they had four females and one male left. The four female pups ran up to me and jumped on my legs with their claws; they were scratching me and biting my hands. In sheer terror, I was thinking, *Please, stop!* They were only eight weeks old and were probably just being puppies, but to me, they just seemed crazy.

In the midst of all the chaos, I looked over and saw a gray blob in the corner. "What's that one?" I asked about the big sleeping ball of a dog.

"Oh, that's the biggest of the litter. He's a male, and nobody wants him because he's so big. He's never going to be a show dog," she explained. That was just fine with me, as I didn't want a show dog anyway.

By now my legs were bleeding, and the woman said, "Here, let me help you," as she shooed the females away. I walked over to the gray ball, and he stood up. He was so cute, this puppy, because his ears hit the ground when he walked. I've read that the Weimaraner ear, at eight weeks of age, is the size it's going to be when they're an adult. He was precious.

So he came lumbering over. He smelled me, looked around, and then lumbered back to his spot in the corner and lay down again, like he could take me or leave me. I said, "That one!"

Mike was pulling on my shirt, "Pam, let's not make a decision yet. We still have to see the Vizslas." Always with the common sense in the family, he was right. So we took an interesting ride across town to a house in Central Phoenix.

This family must have had twelve Vizsla puppies, and they made the Weimaraner pups look calm. These were like little beasts on speed. As we drove up, the owner was feeding them scrambled eggs. There was stuff everywhere, and it was an utter nightmare. We walked up, and immediately the puppies were doing the same thing to me as the Weimaraners had: scratching, scratching, scratching. Things were utterly berserk, so it was a very short visit. I told Mike, "I've gotta get out of here!"

I don't know if the woman even realized we had left, because we just got in the car and drove away — it was so traumatic. "I only wanted a puppy!" I was sitting in the car, breathing heavily, when I looked at Mike, and he looked at me. We didn't say a word. I picked up my cell phone. "Can we come see that male Weimaraner puppy again?"

"I didn't know if you'd be back or not," the woman's kind voice said.

I said, "Yes — but could you get the other ones out of the way before we get there?"

We went back, and he was exactly the same. He was just this soul — like an old soul in a puppy. And I felt like he came to me. I felt like he was mine. I fell in love.

Mike and I took him outside for a little walk — thank God, because he had a big poop, and that would have happened in the car! Would not have been the best way to start things off. After he was done taking care of his business, we brought him home. I held him in my arms as Mike drove, smelling his soft fur. I was lost in puppy breath. I felt like I'd found a soul mate in an animal. That's how it felt to me. Little did I know that this big soft bundle of gray fluff would grow into the dog who would start a revolution.

CHAPTER TWO

Farewell to "Dog Eat Dog"

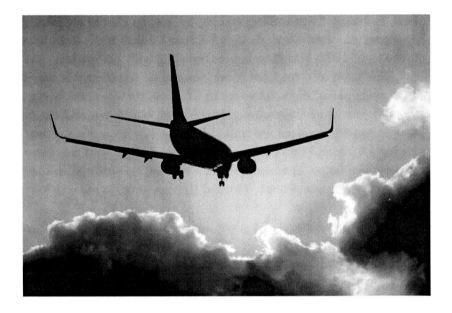

I was home changing suitcases. In those days, I changed suitcases like some people change clothes. I was running the pet and veterinary divisions of the company I worked for, overseeing six regional managers all across the United States, which meant I was traveling heavily. I was home, on average, three days a month. Thing is, this was everything I'd always thought I wanted as a young girl. I had dreamed of being a successful leader in business, but I'd never envisioned the white picket fence and 2.2 kids. I saw the husband, maybe, and definitely the dogs, but I didn't see any of the rest of it. Now, here I was with a high-level career and essentially everything I had ever wanted, yet it was starting to feel empty. I began to find myself wondering, *This is my life?*

A chance meeting in early 1997 brought things to a head. I was at Phoenix Sky Harbor Airport, leaving home to head back to Chicago, dragging my luggage through the terminal and feeling pretty sorry for myself. I looked at the list of departing flights and hiked to Gate A14. Across the aisle, at Gate A16, I saw people coming off their plane, all of them appearing to have smiling faces, as if they might be happily arriving home or coming to visit relatives. Then, in the middle of all the smiling, happy faces, I saw my husband, Mike, emerging from the same plane. Suddenly I was smiling and happy, too, so glad to see him. The happiness was short-lived, though, because I didn't really even have a chance to talk with him since he was traveling with a coworker.

Mike's job also required a fair amount of traveling. He was the CFO for a homebuilder's Active Adult Division. He was a numbers guy, and while our work lives were very different, our values and views of life were exactly the same. He smiled when he saw me and came over to give me a big hug. I think for a brief moment he thought I was there to welcome him home. Then he looked down, saw my suitcase, and knew I was on my way out of town. Two sad ships passing on the way to baggage claim.

I said, "I've gotta go. My plane … I have to board."

He said, "I'll see ya…"

I waved and boarded my plane. I had a window seat, I'll never forget — and found myself thinking, *What is this? This is my life? What am I doing?* Feelings of loneliness and emptiness engulfed me. During that long plane ride, I had time to seriously consider what was driving me to be so successful. What is success anyway? Money? Power? A corner office? I felt as though I had reached the pinnacle of my career, and I looked down at a panoramic view of my life. I had worked hard to crash through the glass ceiling, but all that had really given me was a splitting headache.

My decision to work so hard was not about money or material things. I believe a person needs meaningful work, but somehow I'd begun to lose the meaning — the "why" in why I work. The plane landed in Chicago, and it was back to work, work, work, same as always. But my chance meeting with Mike was a turning point that really made me start thinking.

Not long after that, I was browsing a bookstore during one of my innumerable trips when I saw a book titled, *Why Women Work*. I said to myself, "I'm going to buy that book!" Because I truly didn't know why I was working anymore.

Though we made a very comfortable living, Mike and I had saved most of our money because all we did was work; we were never home to spend it. I remember reading in *Why Women Work* how so much of our identity is wrapped up in what we do. I began to wonder, *Who am I without my career?* I had invested my whole self into my work and now defined myself through it. We hear that about men all the time, but you didn't hear it so much about women back then.

During the next year, I read many books about finding your authentic self; I was on a journey of self-exploration. It wasn't necessarily an on-purpose journey, but trying to figure out what I really wanted for my life was what fed my soul. What I was doing, what life meant, what was really important. That panoramic view of my life really shook me up, because I never expected to get to the top and then find myself thinking, *So this is it? What a sham!*

One thing I felt was a strong desire to be connected to my community. Up to this point, my "local" newspaper had been *USA Today*, because that was what showed up outside my hotel room every morning. I never even saw our local paper, *The Arizona Republic*. I was so disconnected from my community, and I wanted the chance to make a difference … somehow.

I recall mentioning to Mike, here and there, "You know, I'm really not happy. I'm never home. I feel so disconnected, and all the traveling is beginning to lose its glamour and appeal." Right around that time, the company I worked for was going through a merger with another pharmaceutical giant. Mergers are never easy, and this one was no fun. The process took its toll on staff at every level, and it probably sped up my decision to leave.

One morning, mid-merger, I went for a run. Climbing up the front steps, I sat in the rocking chair on my porch — our house faced the nature preserve — and looked at the mountain. Then I took a deep breath, picked up the phone, and called the president of my company: "I'm done."

"Excuse me?" she said. "Are you crazy?"

I repeated, "I'm done. I'm really done. I've been traveling for fifteen years. I don't even know my next-door neighbors. And I need the second part of my life to start now. I need to do something different."

I hung up the phone and went inside. I found Mike in the bathroom shaving, and I just stared at him. He looked at me and asked, "What are you doing? Are you okay?" I must have looked like I'd seen a ghost, or something equally scary.

"I just resigned."

"Ohhhhh…" was all he said. He knew I'd been thinking about it, but I hadn't told him when I was going to do it — probably because I didn't know until the moment I did it. But he was so supportive. He always said to me, "Do what you need to do. Whatever makes you happy. I'm good." Because in his heart, he has always wanted me to be happy. At that moment, I was just glad he didn't cut himself with the razor.

Fortunately, money wasn't going to be an issue. We'd always been very conservative with our money. Most childless couples in their late thirties, early forties, would have been living in an oversized mansion — but for what? To impress our friends? To keep up with the Joneses? We neither wanted nor needed that. So I knew I could make the decision to resign and that things would still be fine for our family. At that time, we had two cats, and they're cheap to feed — oh, but that was soon to change, too! Now I was in transition mode.

My company had a nice send-off party for me. I flew up to Chicago, and it was very cordial with all the formalities of seeing off a corporate higher-up. But at the end of the day, when you leave Corporate America, they say, "See ya! Bye!" Not that I felt bad for one moment. On the contrary, I felt liberated and free. Not knowing what was coming next didn't bother me in the least. The sense of peace I felt surprised me a bit, as I'd thought my identity was so wrapped up in my job. I could see now that all my insecurities were unfounded. I was Pam Gaber, CEO of Me!

CHAPTER THREE

Pam, the Volunteer

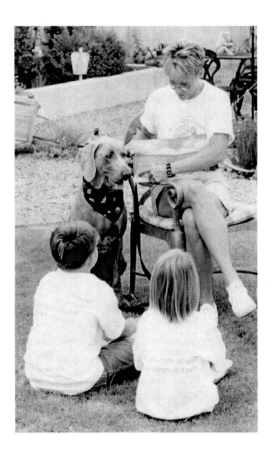

Over the next several months, I began to feel alive again. I noticed the sunbeams coming through the kitchen window and how my chubby kitty would stretch out and enjoy the moment. I noticed how the desert smelled after a light rain. But most importantly, I noticed myself and my growing desire to connect with my community.

One morning, about halfway through my daily run, I had this overwhelming desire to do something ... anything ... for my community. By now, I had gotten to know a couple of my neighbors, and I knew they were people who knew people. So I thought, *Hmmm. What if Mike and I have a Christmas party at our home?* We had never had done anything like that before, and it was an exciting idea for me. But I didn't want hostess gifts for myself — I wanted to help the community. If only I could figure out a way to combine the party with making a difference. Then it crossed my mind that people would still want to bring something — so I decided to ask them to bring something that could be donated to people in need. I realize now that this idea was neither new nor unique, but for me at the time, it was huge.

I didn't know what types of items to ask the guests to bring — maybe something to help women or children? I felt really clueless. It occurred to me that I could call the police and ask for suggestions ... or I could call the fire department. Given that the fire department had a reputation for much more interesting men, and far more handsome, I called them.

I connected with Captain John Dean on the first try, and he turned out to be exactly the person I needed to speak with. He told me that his firehouse held a toy drive every year for the Crisis Nursery, and that the firemen delivered the collected toys to the children at their annual holiday party. Not only that, but the toys were delivered by Santa, via helicopter! How fun is that? Of course, my first question was, "What's the Crisis Nursery?" Captain Dean told me it was a safe haven for abused and neglected children who had been removed from the care of their parents. Those words hit me right in the heart. I said, "Tell me how I can help."

Captain Dean told me that they had already collected a lot of toys, but that these kids always needed shoes. Casual shoes, not patent leather Mary Janes — just plain, old running-around shoes. I loved that idea, because when I was a kid, getting new sneakers was always the highlight of my summer. When I got new sneakers, I swear I could run faster! I ran like the wind in my new shoes, the fastest kid on earth! So I thought shoes were a great idea.

I sent out invitations to about a hundred people, asking each of them to bring a pair of brand new canvas shoes for kids, ages ten years and younger. The party was a success, and these people, none of whom

I knew that well, didn't just bring one pair each. They brought two, three, five pairs of shoes. The pile of shoes was so immense that we could hardly see the Christmas tree behind them.

John Dean told me that if I could get a hundred people to attend my party, he would bring the fire truck that night to pick up the shoes, and he would dress up as Santa for the party. I accepted his challenge, as that would certainly be a hit! The clock approached ten, and I saw red flashing lights outside as the fire truck pulled up. The neighbors might have thought I was burning my house down, except that for once, all my neighbors were at my house. Captain Santa Dean came in, handing out candy canes, while the firemen loaded the shoes into the fire truck. There must have been five hundred pairs.

Captain Dean said to me, "You know, Wednesday is the Crisis Nursery Christmas party — the day we'll be delivering the toys and shoes. You *have* to come." I wouldn't have missed it. I could scarcely wait to see the children's eyes light up!

I drove to the nursery with a sense of excitement, wondering what the children would be like. Knowing they were victims of abuse and neglect just broke my heart, but this was an organization that provided a safe place for them. Although I'd never had children of my own, I had always had a soft spot for little people. As I got out of my car, a helicopter was hovering overhead. The children were in the parking lot, jumping up and down, clapping their hands, and shouting "Santa, Santa, Santa!" Just as Captain Dean had promised, Santa was in that helicopter! Made sense, though. This was Arizona where we don't really have sleigh-drawn reindeer. But a helicopter? Amazing!

I was so touched by these little children — in so many ways they looked like regular kids. They were cute and cuddly. But these kids were victims of abuse, neglect, and violence. I'd notice a bruise here and there, and saw that behaviorally they were different. If one child ran into another, rather than saying they were sorry or just ignoring it, they would threaten to fight. Yet in spite of the drama, I was hooked. It really was a beautiful time, and I found myself thinking, *I could get attached to this organization.*

So I began my volunteer career at the Crisis Nursery in Phoenix in early 1998.

GABRIEL'S ANGELS

You might think volunteering came naturally to me, but that was not the case. I came from a family that did not volunteer. Period. I honestly believe that the average high school student has logged more volunteer hours than I had when I first began working at the Crisis Nursery. I guess I was making up for lost time, because I spent a lot of time there. And when I started Gabriel's Angels, I felt a deep sense of obligation to help these children. Until then, I had been unaware that it was our duty to make our community a better place. I hadn't really had a community for fifteen years, so now I had such a compulsion — in a good way — to give back.

During my corporate career, my head was in the sand. I didn't know about domestic violence or child abuse because I chose not to know. I didn't understand how important volunteering is for all segments of a community. But now I believe that if we have the means and the time, it's something everyone should do. It's our duty. At the very least, we can leave the world a bit better than we found it.

Nothing Captain Dean suggested had struck me until he mentioned those little kids and their need for shoes. I firmly believe that of all the people we can help, we most need to help our children, because someday they're going to be us, and they're going to be running the store. They're going to be running an organization. They're going to be running for President.

* * *

I volunteered on what I called "Fun Fridays," frequently accompanying the Crisis Nursery staff when they took the kids on field trips. One of the first people I met during my volunteering was a nice man named Rob, also a volunteer. How great it was for a man to volunteer his time with these special children. In many ways, he was the first truly nice man they had ever met. Little boys would cling to Rob and hang on his every word. But they didn't just hang onto Rob.

The first time we took the kids to the zoo, I was scared because I thought that four adults — of which I was just a helper — and thirteen kids was not a good ratio. Fears preyed on me: *We're gonna lose some kids, and it will be on my watch.* I could just see them climbing into the elephant enclosure, the monkey pen, or the jaguar cage. Or slipping away in the crowd.

What I learned, however, was that these children don't leave you. They become little Velcro people. I was trying to go to the ladies room, and they were literally hanging on me. "Where are you going, Miss Pam? Don't leave, Miss Pam!" Wow! They were so afraid we were going to leave them, because all the adults in their lives had left and not come back. Talk about heartbreaking.

On some Fridays, we would take them to do something simple, like go to the park so they could swing on the swings. My arms used to ache from pushing the swings, but the kids were having so much fun just doing what kids do.

One time, we took them to the Children's Museum. That didn't go so well. The children were, again, doing as children do, which means they were touching everything. It's a *children's* museum, yet there were signs everywhere: DO NOT TOUCH. So, needless to say, we were asked to leave and not to come back.

CHAPTER FOUR

Gabriel's First Year

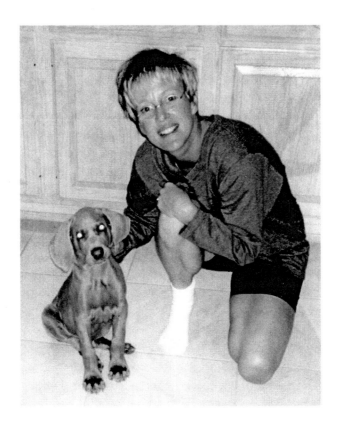

When we brought this puppy home, we had no idea what we were going to name him. We considered all kinds of dog names. Finally my husband said, "Why don't we name him Gabriel?"

After all the other names we'd been considering, that one immediately resonated. I said, "Gabriel. That's a great name. How'd you come up with that?"

"Well," he said, "I want to call him Gabe for short."

"OK. So how'd you come up with that?" Our last name is Gaber. Was there a connection here?

"Well, I want to call him Gabe, because when I played basketball as a teenager, my nickname was ... Gabe."

I promptly looked at my husband and asked him, "So you're naming the dog after *yourself*?!? Clarify! We're naming our puppy after you?"

He nodded sheepishly, "Well, yeah."

"I'm not telling anybody that, ever," I said. I guess, though, it's time for the truth to come out.

And we've always laughed about that. But I loved the name Gabriel and calling him Gabe. I mean, he was eight weeks old and named after an angel. That decision alone contained more than a little irony. But who knew this dog would one day live up to that angelic status, teaching us all to help the kids who most needed us? It was all perfect — it was meant to be.

* * *

Gabriel was about five months old when our vet, Dr. Dean Rice, recommended we get him neutered. But my manly pooch had only one testicle descended. It's a condition called cryptorchidism, actually rather common in purebred dogs. Treating it involves one of two things: you wait for the other testicle to descend, or you go in during the neuter to surgically remove it.

We made the appointment to get him neutered, and Dr. Rice searched for the hidden testicle. Unfortunately, the second testicle was too small and well hidden to be found, so he only got the one he could see. "That poor dog wasn't normal from the beginning," Dr. Rice recently quipped. For perhaps the next three months, I palpated Gabe's abdomen. Finally, I thought I felt a small bump. I took him in, and Dr. Rice agreed. In essence Gabriel was neutered twice!

Right before his second neutering, Gabriel was due to be microchipped. We wanted to make sure he had permanent identification in case he got out and someone found him. Microchipping involves the vet injecting a little seed under the skin which is readable and identifies the dog and its owners. We figured this was a good time to do it, since Gabe was getting his rabies vaccine at the same time.

The projected order was rabies vaccine first, and the microchip would follow. The needle used to administer the rabies vaccine is about the width of a piece of human hair. This tiny little needle is used to inject the vaccine into the muscle of the rear leg. It didn't matter that the needle was nearly invisible — as Dr. Rice gave him the injection, Gabriel started howling and crying like he was being knifed or bludgeoned to death. I don't know, technically, if dogs scream, but the blood-curdling sound was worse than any horror movie I ever saw. Every vet and tech in the hospital came running in, shouting, "What's wrong???"

"I only gave him his rabies shot," Dr. Rice answered. "Seems our Gabriel has a low threshold for pain." While the rabies vaccine needle is tiny, the needle for the microchip insertion is about ten times bigger, so Dr. Rice said, "I think we're just going to put this microchip needle right back in the box, and when we neuter him, we'll go ahead and do the microchip."

* * *

So, there we were, in full-fledged puppydom. To be honest, I hadn't done that much research or reading about the commitment necessary to become the parent of a Weimaraner. I naively thought I could handle any dog. I learned. People still say to me, "Oh, Weimaraner puppies are so cute. We have a two-year-old son and a four-year-old daughter, and we're going to get two Weimies."

I always tell them, "Wait until your children are older." These dogs need an hour a day of exercise. Without exercise, they start to destroy things. They will tear up everything in sight in an effort to get some kind of attention. Much like children, even negative attention is better than no attention at all. Trust me, I know.

Though Gabriel was no ordinary dog, in many ways he was an ordinary puppy. Full of life and energy during the day, at night he was also restless, so I was up every two hours. I even slept on the kitchen floor with him one night. He was out cold, but I was just plain freezing cold — and awake.

Being first-time dog owners, a crate seemed out of the question. We should have listened to our dog owner friends who suggested that we crate train Gabe. Eleven years wiser, I totally agree. He broke down every barrier and gate we put up because he just wanted to be with us — all the time — every living, breathing minute. And I was in heaven.

But active is an understatement. He was a handful. It's amazing that Gabe lived through his first year — and that I lived through it, too. I have a photo of him at about six months, flying through the family room and jumping off the couch. He was a wild child who wanted nothing more than to play. After he ate every dog bed we bought, I knew we needed help.

I located a dog trainer who came to the house to interview us. I was a nervous wreck. What if she would not agree to work with the crazy puppy? We had Gabriel gated in the kitchen when she arrived. She walked in, and BAMM! Down came the gate, and out bounded Gabriel to greet this new friend. She totally ignored him, which initially made him try even harder to get her attention. I thought to myself, *She doesn't like him, and we are going to get fired before we even hire her.* Amazingly, though, he calmed down enough for her to acknowledge his presence, which sent him into another frenzy. She ignored him again. Soon she petted him and spoke quietly. He was soooo good. Mike and I had been doing pretty much everything wrong, and in our human way, were encouraging his crazy behavior. But he was so darned cute.

Trainer Eileen told us that Weimaraners are smart and have high energy. They, like all dogs, need to know who is in charge, which, incidentally and much to Gabriel's surprise, was not him. We were in charge, and we had to start acting like it. She made sense to Mike and me, so we did exactly what she told us to do. Every week Eileen would show up at our house to see the progress Gabriel and I had made. Actually, it was me she was training. Mike designated me the puppy trainer, and if you ask me, he got off easy.

Little by little, Gabriel came around. I remember the day he finally understood what to do when I said "Sit." He sat and looked at me as if to say, "So why weren't you clearer all these weeks? THIS is what you wanted me to do?" When he figured out a treat was part of the deal, he would see me and sit whether or not I commanded him to do so. Of all the pluses of puppy training, one of the biggest is seeing the light bulb go on when they finally understand what you want them to do.

Gabriel and I spent many hours practicing on the volleyball court at the side of our house. He learned to heel, sit, lie down, and stay. He was really quite good. One day, out of nowhere, he freaked out because he noticed the pool pump. "The pool pump?" I asked. "That pump has been there every time we've been out here!" But I took immense joy in watching his mind grow as he noticed things that had been there the entire time.

* * *

One thing to keep in mind as you're training a dog is that these animals so want to please, but they don't always know what you want. And I think that can become frustrating for people. They say things like, "Well, my dog can't sit. He can't be a therapy dog — my dog doesn't sit."

The truth is, it doesn't matter if your dog is a Maltese or a Great Dane — all their brains work the same way, and they can't do it if they don't know what you want. I learned to be a better pet owner once I understood that innately, Gabriel just wanted to please me. The mistakes were my human errors; it wasn't his fault he didn't know what I wanted from him.

The biggest mistake dog owners make is looking at things from a human perspective. The problem is, we don't really think like dogs. Early on, I would humanize Gabe. I would think, *Oh, he did this because I did that*, when in reality, the two were very rarely tied to each other. I do believe, however, that animals have memory. I've heard it said that if you don't catch them in the act of tearing apart the dog bed, it doesn't do any good. I disagree, because on more than one occasion, I walked into the house to find my big gray dog hiding behind the chair, as if to say, "Hi. And no, I didn't do it."

"Really? How interesting, since you are the only dog here!" They do know because they have memory.

* * *

Initially, I put in the minimum training time to keep Gabe successful. I always wanted his training sessions to end on a high note. For example, if I was going to have him stay, I would move back a foot or so, return, and say "Good boy!" Then I would back up one-and-a-half feet, and if he stood up, it was owner error. I would do one foot again so

I could make Gabe successful, which built confidence in him.

When I was training Gabriel, I started with two-minute sessions, twice a day. By the time we finished, I was allotting ten minutes, twice a day. That's really all it takes. Once you go past the ten-minute mark, you start to lose them, especially the puppies. It's all about positive reinforcement and being very consistent.

One thing I will say about our relationship with Gabriel is that I was the pain-in-the-neck mom, disciplinarian, and Chief Enforcement Officer. Mike was in charge of treats, swimming, and all things fun! So needless to say, I had my training challenges. I wondered at times if Gabriel liked Mike best.

* * *

As a puppy, Gabriel wasn't interested in fetching a ball. So I went out of my way — I went OUT of my way — to teach him, because I always thought I would love to have a dog that would bring the ball back. It was my dream. I'd throw the ball, and he'd bring it back — it would be a real bonding experience. You've heard the saying, "Be careful what you wish for"?

When Gabriel was about four months old, I bought a big yellow tennis ball. I showed it to him and threw it across the yard. "Go get it, Gabe!" I would yell. "Come on, Gabriel. Go get the ball."

He'd look at me as if to say, "I ain't gonna go get that ball. You think it's such a good idea, you go get the ball." So I would get the ball, show it to him, and throw it again. He would stare at me and walk away. I was heartbroken, thinking I would never have a dog that would fetch, and thus no bonding.

I kept trying, continuing to throw that darned ball every night. Mike would come out with us and retrieve the ball so that Gabriel could have a visual of what we were trying to get him to do. Funny, a retrieving husband — not exactly what I had in mind. Finally, one day when Gabriel was about six months old, the light bulb flashed, and he looked at me as if to say, "Oh, I get it. If I bring it back, you're going to throw it again. You humans have some weird need to throw that ball. But I'll go along with it. I will bring it back so you can play your silly game." Maybe he thought he was helping me exercise.

But then things began to change. Gabriel delighted in retrieving the ball, so much so that we created a monster. A ball-aholic. His non-work life revolved around fetching. He retrieved the ball from dry land or the pool. We'd come home from visiting with the kids, and he'd bat at the plastic bin that held the balls. He'd bat and bat and bat at it. Finally he'd just stare at us like, "Give me the ball, or someone is going to get hurt."

Mike would just laugh, "So why'd you work so hard to get him to fetch?" For the next eleven-and-a-half years, either Mike or I had to throw his beloved blue ball every single day, because he loved it so much. Later, though, when he was sick, I said to Mike, "I will never complain again about throwing that blue ball." And when he got better, we did throw the ball again.

* * *

As Gabriel grew, he continued to be challenging because he was so smart. You couldn't make one mistake, as he would put two and two together quite nicely. One day, he kept scratching the pantry door, I suspect because he wanted a cookie. I was working on the computer and really didn't want to be bothered, so I got up, went into the pantry, and gave him a cookie. Immediately, he was like, "Ohhhh ... that's how you get a cookie!" So he kept scratching the door incessantly. I only did it the one time, and he caught onto it. *I must be more careful*, I thought.

So puppyhood with Gabriel was filled with training, because I knew that he was going to be a big dog. If we were going to walk down the street, I didn't want him telling me which way we would go. And I certainly didn't want him jumping on people. I wanted a dog with manners. As he matured, reaching six, seven, eight months, he loved everyone. Gabriel could intuitively tell when someone had had a bad day. Not just with Mike and me, but with anybody. He had what I call "the gift." He would go over and nuzzle someone, as if he knew they were having a tough time.

CHAPTER FIVE

The Christmas Visit

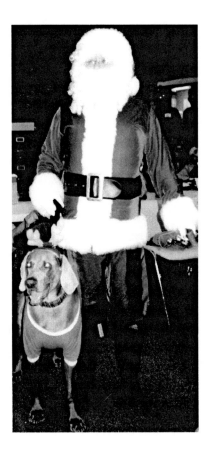

My volunteer work at Crisis Nursery coincided with Gabriel's first year of life. The Friday after we adopted him, I told the kids, "I just got a new puppy!"

"What did you name him?" they asked excitedly.

"We named him Gabriel."

The next Friday, they asked, "Miss Pam, how's Gabriel?" I told them that Gabriel had his first bath.

The kids' eyes were wide as I told them how Gabriel had been in the tub, shaking soap and water everywhere. I described how I dried his soft fur and how good he smelled afterwards. "What did he do next?" they asked.

"He fell asleep in my arms."

"Awww," the kids responded.

Every time I visited the nursery, they asked about Gabriel and wanted to see pictures, "What did Gabriel do this week? What did he do?"

"Gabriel ate my shoe."

"Wow — Gabriel ate your shoe. Did you hit him?" one tiny guy asked. In that moment, I was reminded that this little boy was a victim of abuse and neglect.

"Oh, no," I said. "I just threw away the other shoe. So now I don't have those shoes anymore. Gabriel didn't mean to eat my shoe. I left it on the bedroom floor, and he thought it was a toy." I told them about the times Gabriel ate his bed and tore up the outdoor drip system. They were always interested in hearing how, when Gabriel was challenging, I never hurt him. I now realize that those little stories were lessons about compassion for these kids. They learned that Gabriel was a member of our family, and in my family we did not resolve issues with violence.

I began taking a little album with photos of Gabe to share with the kids. It had various pictures of Gabriel at home sleeping, eating, and playing. The pictures illustrated for the children that Gabriel was part of our family and was always treated as such. One photo was of a huge, beautiful lake with a tiny dot — Gabriel fetching a stick — right in the middle. I would ask, "Where is Gabriel?" And they would point their tiny little fingers right at the dot.

* * *

Since I'd been sharing all the details of Gabriel's first year with the children, I wanted them to meet him. After all, they had been bonding with an animal they had never met. The perfect opportunity presented itself, so I seized the moment. Marsha Porter was the Executive Director of the Crisis Nursery, and I needed her permission to carry out my plan. "I know you're having your annual Christmas party in December. And I came last year — without a dog. How about this year I bring Gabriel dressed as Rudolph so the kids can finally meet him?"

She looked at me and said, "That's interesting."

Interesting? I thought. *That certainly doesn't mean no.*

Off I went to our local doggie boutique, where I purchased a pair of doggie antlers, a "Just Call Me Rudolph" t-shirt, and a big jingle bell collar. Quite honestly, I was amazed at all the Christmas regalia available for dogs at that store. That night, Gabe modeled his reindeer outfit for Mike. I thought he might mind the costume, but Gabriel was beaming, as if to say, "Look at me!" He strutted his stuff down our hallway and around the living room.

The day of the party, we arrived at the Crisis Nursery, and Gabriel jumped out of the car in full reindeer regalia, anxious to greet the children. We walked into the nursery. The children noticed me first, and then their eyes lit up like Christmas trees when they saw Gabriel. At first they were a little confused about whether it was a dog at the end of the leash, or a real reindeer. Some were quite hesitant. "Hi, everyone," I said. "I brought Gabriel to meet you, and he decided to get dressed up like one of Santa's reindeer. Would you like to pet him?"

After volunteering with these children every Friday for a year, I had gotten to know them pretty well, but that day they were different. They did not display any anger or violent tendencies; they were simply kind and loving toward Gabriel. They would gently pat his head and hug him. They carefully took his velvety ear and touched it against their cheeks. The nursery became an oasis of peace and serenity. And the only difference that day was the presence of a gentle gray dog.

I remember one little boy who was about five years old, with dark hair and a Spiderman t-shirt. He had just been admitted to the nursery and was in his room crying, uninterested in coming to the party. Even when a child is removed from a violent home and taken to a safe haven, he's scared to death because he doesn't know what safety is. Familiar violence feels safer than a peaceful place with strangers. Though the nursery accepted children from birth to age ten, most of these kids seemed to be between four and six years of age. It makes sense, because stress often elevates during the holidays, and it's generally the little ones who get pulled from the home because they're just not safe there.

But this little guy kept peeking around the corner to see Gabriel, and before long, he came out and draped his arms around Gabriel's neck and buried his head in the soft fur. The boy not only stopped crying, but began to smile and laugh. Gabriel's eyes were a limitless pool of understanding that day. Soon the line for photos with "Rudolph" was longer than the line for photos with Santa!

We all stood in amazement at how Gabriel, without any effort on his part, was reaching these children in a way no human had been able to. It was as if we were watching a movie unravel its plot. Gabriel and I were preparing to leave the party when the shelter director said to me, "I don't know what happened here today, but would you bring Gabriel back?" Wow, really? I felt like someone had just told me my child was a genius. I checked Gabe's calendar, which happened to be free — so I said YES!

As we got in the car to head home, I sensed that something profound had happened. I had witnessed Gabriel reach those children like no person seemed able to. Normally angry, impatient, scared kids had been only kind and loving. I was deeply moved by all of it. I remember thinking that something magical had happened in that nursery, and I could either do something to create more magic, or I could do nothing and let it end there. I decided in that moment that I was going to do something. I just didn't know quite what.

CHAPTER SIX

The Birth of Gabriel's Angels

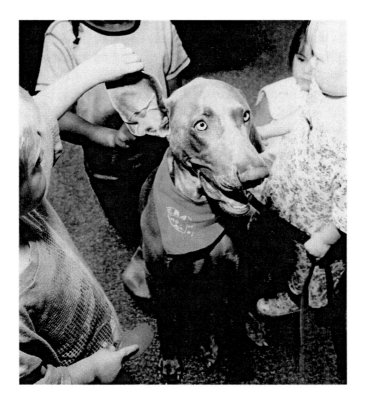

After the kids' remarkable response to Gabe at the Christmas party, I made the decision that I had to do something more, whether it was just Gabriel and I visiting children, or something bigger than that. The best idea seemed to be joining a group of pet therapy teams that were already doing what I wanted to do, visiting children in crisis, but I soon found out there weren't any programs like that — not in Arizona, or anywhere in the country.

I did some research online and found the Delta Society, a national organization that registers people and their pets as therapy teams. The dog and its handler go through a course known as the Pet Partner Program. According to Jan Hutchinson, a former Delta evaluator and instructor from Tucson, once a dog is registered through Delta Society, it can visit old people, children, almost anyone. "The sky's the limit — as long as you can find a facility that allows and understands the benefit of bringing in animals to visit with people."

I found a local Delta evaluator named Diane Decker and learned from her that Gabriel needed basic obedience training, which of course we had already done. Beyond that, though, he needed to be exposed to many different scenarios, as the testing would require that. I decided to take Gabriel to my local PetSmart store and walk around. He did pretty well, considering all the distractions ... until I took him to see the automatic doors at the entrance. The first time the automatic door opened, he almost flew out of his skin. So I thought to myself, *Okay, we're going to have to sit here awhile.* By the fiftieth time the door opened, he was perfectly calm, even looking at me as if to say, "What? This is no big deal!"

I took him lots of places and exposed him to many different things, so anything we encountered became simply just another new thing. In working with children, especially the children at the Crisis Nursery, there is always something new, so the more exposure to new things, the better.

* * *

To hear Diane tell it now, it took her quite a while to understand the benefit of the program I was trying to create. "Though I thought it was a good idea," Diane says, "I thought it was a huge undertaking. I had just become a Delta evaluator, so at the time, I didn't really see the broad scope of how influential these dogs could be. My own dog and I eventually became a Gabriel's Angels therapy team, but at this point, I thought, 'Nice dog, and Pam's a wonderful person,' but I just didn't see it. It seemed like it was just going to be kids petting dogs. It wasn't until I was visiting with my dog in children's wards — which I hadn't done before — that I saw the huge relief just the silliness of a dog can make for the kids, the sheer happiness a dog can bring."

When Diane began working with Gabe and me, she heard my stories of how Gabriel was able to get the kids to talk about some pretty awful things that had happened to them. Even in telling these horror stories, they felt okay afterward, because Gabriel was there. She seemed most surprised to learn that if Gabriel hadn't been there, the kids would have kept the violence bottled up inside, never saying anything. "And then I started thinking that dogs can really make a difference in these centers," Diane says. "There's so much chaos going on there anyway. To give them something else to focus on — like a dog that can absorb all of that for the hour he's there — that is an amazing feat."

As good a therapy dog as Gabriel turned out to be, he wasn't exactly a star student. In the beginning, he could barely sit still, although you could tell he really wanted to. But he was a youthful Waimaraner, so he was like, "Sitting still? But what's it for?" The whole concept of the thirty-minute Delta evaluation seemed to be more than he could handle. But I would say to Diane, "Work with me. I'm getting him there."

I continued to share stories with Diane about Gabe's work, and I started to meet people who wanted their dogs to become therapy dogs, so I sent them to her for evaluation, excitedly telling her, "I found more people for my program!"

"After a while," Diane recalls, "I started seeing that this pet therapy for abused kids was really working — this was really something. And then those newly minted pet therapy teams stated coming back with their own stories and pictures of what they were doing or little cards the kids would send them or letters of thanks from the moms." I think by this point, she knew we were here to stay.

The test that Gabriel — and all Delta therapy dogs — had to take is based on the Canine Good Citizen® test (CGC), which was outlined by the American Kennel Club (AKC). Delta Society used that as its starting point and then added more parameters, including things like requiring that the dog be exposed to wheelchairs, loud noises, and lots of petting, situations it might encounter in a group setting. Also, the dog has to be able to walk well on a leash. It may be the nicest dog in the world, but we can't have a dog that pulls. It has to stay with its owner. Delta Society is looking for a team spirit between the dog and its handler, regardless of whether it's for Gabriel's Angels or for therapy work in a hospital, hospice, school, or prison.

It was Diane who helped me understand how important it was for Gabe to know the difference between hanging out at home and putting on his vest to go see the kids. "Your dog needs to be with you and understand that they're doing a job," Diane says. "They're not there just to look cute or get lots of attention. They're there to work."

Another piece of the Delta training is knowing that if something drops on the ground — like a pill in a hospital or a crayon in a school setting — the dog will leave it alone and not go chasing after it. That was Gabriel's worst fault. We always joked about it, because Diane would always bring out a ball, and I would plead, "Diane, anything but a ball!"

Though it was a struggle for both of us, eventually Gabriel learned to leave the ball alone. But you could tell that every inch of his being was like, "Ball? Ball!"

Perhaps the biggest thing Delta evaluators watch for is the teamwork and camaraderie between the human and the dog. Does the handler know where their dog is? Will the handler always keep their dog safe? Is the handler always willing to work through new things with their dog, especially in the beginning? "My goal is always to see a good team," Diane explains, "not necessarily to see the dog that sits still the best, because that's not really the point.

"Safety is a big issue, too. If I thought my dog were in any sort of danger, I would move him out of the way — not just let it happen. But a lot of people aren't proactive that way, because they're just not aware. They're so taken by the fact that their dog is cute — and being such a helpful, productive good citizen — that they forget that they need to be involved in the work, too. Handlers need to be in sync with their dogs — that's probably the most important thing."

One question I asked Diane early on was, "How do I know Gabriel is enjoying the work?"

Her answer was, "If you put that vest on and his personality changes in a positive way, then he's excited to go. You know that he wants to do this." The interesting thing is that the dogs that enjoy the work the most tend to be the best therapy dogs. "They might not be the best team in the world from a technical standpoint," Diane says, "but they love what they're doing, so they do it well."

* * *

Gabriel and I got registered as a therapy team in 2000. A couple of friends told me they had great dogs and were interested in helping out, so they got their dogs registered, too. It was August 2000, and we had a total of three teams visiting the Crisis Nursery. That was all I envisioned at the time, our small group of therapy teams visiting children in crisis. Then my community newspaper, the *Ahwatukee Foothills News*, contacted me because they wanted to do an article on Gabriel's work with the children, and I thought, *Well, that is really nice.* Ahwatukee is a pretty small community, and they had found out about us via word of mouth.

The reporter interviewed me over the phone and sent a photographer to accompany Gabriel and me on our next visit. The photographer understood that the children did not have photo releases, so he had to get his shots without any faces. He snapped away, the bulbs flashing constantly. Still, Gabriel sat with the children, ignoring the camera. It was as if he had been in that situation a million times before.

The paper was delivered to my driveway, and guess who was on the front page! Gabriel was front and center, with the side view of a little girl holding up his ear and looking inside. The headline read, "Special Dogs Make a Difference in Children's Lives."

A few days later, the phone rang, and the caller identified himself as a reporter from a local television station. I froze, as images from my past career in the pharmaceutical/chemical industry immediately came to mind. In that job, a phone call from the media usually was not a good thing. When the media called, we were instructed to say only, "No comment," and forward them to Media Relations. I quickly remembered this was another time and place, gathering my composure and cracking a joke: "Oh, you're not outside my door with cameras, are you? Like *Sixty Minutes?*"

The reporter sounded amused, "That's not even our station!" He went on to introduce himself and explain that one of the vice presidents from Channel 3 had read the article about Gabriel in the Ahwatukee paper and wanted him to do a story on "that dog and that girl." Then it hit me. He was calling me to do a television news story about Gabe!

I said, "Can you hold a minute, Wade?"

Mike was standing there and asked, "Who is it?"

I put my hand over the receiver. "It's Channel 3, and they want to do a story on my program!"

And Mike, the good old finance guy who always sees everything in black and white, said, "But you don't have a program! At least nothing formal."

The thought ran through my head, *Thanks for the boost of confidence,* but I said, "I know!"

I picked up the phone again and asked Wade, "Well, what do you have in mind?"

"We want to film Gabriel working with the kids."

I asked Wade if I could get back to him at the end of the week so I could check with the nursery about filming and find out what other logistics would be involved. In addition, I knew Gabriel was still new enough at this whole visiting process that we could definitely use more time getting to know the children. The Crisis Nursery granted permission for the segment to be filmed, as there were several children who did have photo releases. Then Gabe and I changed our routine to begin visiting every day for a week so we could get some more experience.

Finally, the day of filming arrived. I was so nervous. After they'd gotten all the footage they wanted, Wade interviewed me, and I don't even remember what I said. When the segment aired, I was so excited. It's funny to watch the piece now, because I can see how huge Gabriel's eyes were and how nervous I was. It wasn't until I saw how loving the children were that I liked the segment. It was so organic, in that nothing was staged.

I look back now at the times when we've had media accompany us to a visit. What transpires between a therapy dog and a child is so pure and so natural; it is never made up, and it's never choreographed or rehearsed. The interaction between Gabriel and his kids always unfolded so beautifully on tape. Over the years, I also learned to be authentic and calm for the cameras.

* * *

I was concerned that the children might miss us once we'd finished filming and stopped visiting every day, but I found that they easily settled back into a weekly schedule. Much later, Gabe and I were visiting weekly when the media came to do another story. The reporter asked one little boy named Aaron, "What do you like most about Gabriel coming to visit you?"

They put the microphone to Aaron's mouth, and he said, "I love Gabriel because he comes every day." So there you have it — though we clearly saw the kids only weekly, Aaron thought Gabriel visited every day. But that's just life from a kid's perspective. Children simply don't perceive time the same way as adults do. I think kids live in time that isn't guarded like it is once we grow up.

Regarding the optimal frequency of visits, I do believe that if some is good, more is better. A crucial element in our program is the consistency of the team visits. We can't just show up once and then not show up again, because many of these children are just waiting for one of us to mess up; they are so conditioned not to trust adults. They are waiting to be proven right in their belief that trust will inevitably lead to disappointment. But we break that mold by continuing to come back regularly. We never want them to say, "Well, the dog dumped on me, too, just like every adult dumped on me." That consistency is absolutely essential.

* * *

The phone began to ring. Domestic violence shelters, homeless shelters, other crisis nurseries, and group homes all wanted to know if a therapy dog could come to visit their kids. It makes sense now, but at the time, it was an unanticipated challenge. I decided to fill the obvious need and applied for my 501(c)(3) designation. Today, ten years later, we have more than one hundred fifty therapy teams healing more than 13,000 children in crisis each year.

Our pet therapy program grew by word of mouth. We began at Crisis Nursery, which had a preschool that we started visiting, and then the word just began to spread. The agencies speak to each other, but I also did some outreach within the community. I asked the Crisis Nursery, "Where else could we provide pet therapy?" I would learn about a crisis nursery on the east side, and I would reach out to them. All the agencies were so receptive to having a therapy dog visit. It was probably fifty-fifty then, half outreach and half organizations being referred to us. We still continue our outreach efforts, as there could be a group home we've never heard of. We are always mining it. But the big ones, all the domestic violence shelters and homeless shelters — we've worked with all of them.

We also began to get calls from our southern neighbors in Tucson. We were thrilled to expand and have grown to more than forty therapy teams in Southern Arizona. Our most recent growth has been into Northern Arizona, where we have recently begun to recruit therapy teams.

* * *

Besides being a Delta evaluator and instructor, Jan Hutchinson was also a pet therapy volunteer. She started out in the pet therapy world visiting nursing homes with her dog, Annie. She was also visiting a state juvenile corrections facility. At the midpoint in Annie's career, they tried visiting hospitals, but Annie didn't care for that population. However, the hospital coordinator introduced Jan to Casa de los Niños, Tucson's largest crisis nursery.

"We hadn't been volunteering for very long," Jan says, "when I got the news that an organization from Phoenix would be taking over handling all the pet therapy for Casa de los Niños. 'Phoenix?!' I thought. 'Excuse me. What does a Phoenix organization know about the needs of the kids in a Tucson crisis nursery?' The organization, of course, was Gabriel's Angels. I went to the website right away, and saw that their teams were registered with Delta Society, so I knew they were at least on the right track." Jan now heads the Gabriel's Angels Tucson office.

Jan views her volunteers much the same way that I do. "It's like we tell people, to do this kind of work, you have to have a lot of energy and you have to especially care for these kids. A lot of people can't do this kind of work. They ask, 'Don't you get depressed working around these abused and neglected kids? Doesn't it get you down?' And the answer is, 'No!' I really, really don't, because I believe we're making a difference. When I visit them, I don't know their story and I don't know what went on with them. All I know is that when I bring my dog in to see them, they're happy — and this is a good feeling. It's a good thing to do."

She adds, "Some people ultimately can't do it because it requires a lot of energy and flexibility, in terms of dealing with changing situations. Things like facilities' changing budgets, or the facility forgetting that you're coming. But you have to focus on the fact that it's all about the kids. It's not about you and what you require of this facility. You're there for the kids.

"The volunteers who do the best just go with the flow. We've lost some volunteers who say, 'This isn't for me — I need things a little more structured.' It's not that our visits are unstructured. We come at the same time every week. But the children's circumstances change. Sometimes there are a lot of kids; other times there are just a couple of kids. And you have to learn how to deal with it."

* * *

Marsha Porter and I have become good friends since our accidental discovery of the power of pet therapy at that Christmas party all those years ago.

"I think the reason the pet therapy works," Marsha says, "is that the kids are pretty wary of most adults. These four-legged creatures create a phenomenal experience for all of us." Marsha continues, "From an organizational standpoint, the work Gabriel's Angels does is such a contribution to our ongoing programs. The therapy teams bring balance to a sometimes chaotic and rocky situation. It's really sweet to watch, as the children refer to them as 'my team.' They're never 'our team' — they're 'my team.' So they really do connect.

"We continue to see the therapy teams' self-control, empathy, and unconditional love translate with these kids. The kids always knew it was Thursday because Pam and Gabe were going to come. It was very important to them to know that in one week, the team would come back. One area of progress we've been able to measure is the kids' ability to anticipate. They've also learned to overcome their need for immediate gratification and developed the skill of delayed gratification. Some of the children have a tendency to become overstimulated. But after a couple weeks, even those who hang back at first end up settling down and developing the skills of self-control and exploration.

"There's no question that we see Gabriel's Angels as an integral part of our program. Things like traveling petting zoos are entertaining, but these therapy teams are truly impacting the kids in ways that show results. We've partnered with other organizations, but none has had the impact that Gabriel's Angles has." What Marsha doesn't say is that it's these organizations' willingness to bring us in that is equally essential in the success of our teams.

CHAPTER SEVEN

Life with Gabriel

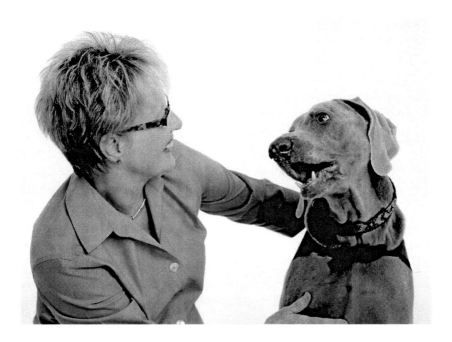

When we brought Gabriel home, he was about fourteen pounds; as an adult, he got up to eighty-nine pounds. I'd always laugh when I saw a Chihuahua, thinking to myself, *Gabriel was that size in the womb!*

He ate a lot of food because he was so active, more than I expected to feed him, actually. Because he had digestion problems, we put him on a totally raw diet, which was really good for him. We also gave him vegetables; he particularly loved broccoli. One time when he wasn't feeling well, he ate all the dog food, but left the broccoli in a ring around his bowl.

Gabe was obviously going to be a big guy, so when we first brought him home, I carried him a lot because I knew the chance to do so would pass quickly. In fact, we'd had him for just a couple weeks, and he was already getting too heavy for me to pick up.

One beautiful February morning, I took my mom and dad on a short hike with Gabriel. He was walking on his little leash when he suddenly tripped and fell into a crevice. His foot slid perfectly into the small niche in the rocks. Immediately, he held up his paw and looked at me with his big blue eyes. Terrified that he might have broken his leg, I carried him down the mountain and all the way home, about two miles. By the time we got there, my arms ached from his weight.

We got into the backyard and I gingerly lowered him to the ground, still frightened that his leg was really hurt. He started walking around the yard, perfectly fine, as if to say, "You didn't have to carry me the *whole* way." *Sure*, I thought. *But that's not how you were acting when you were holding out your delicate little paw, now was it?*

That was the start of Gabriel's love affair with hiking. We'd go out and I would let him off the leash so he could do some investigating. One day, we approached what looked like a little rise in our path. Gabe ran up the berm and over the other side, disappearing from sight. From my vantage point, I couldn't tell if it was a two-foot drop or a hundred-foot drop. I ran toward the spot where he'd disappeared, screaming, "Gabriel!" I pictured him falling hundreds of feet into a gully. I looked over the berm, holding my breath. It turned out to be about a six-foot slide — that's all. Gabriel was just standing there, looking at me like I had gone crazy.

Gabriel and I shared our love of the desert, hiking a couple times a week. It's amazing how, with their huge dog feet, they can still scurry up a hill. I always found myself clambering just to keep up. He would look back at me, as if to say, "Come on! Hurry!" I loved to hide from him when he got too far ahead of me. I'd hide behind a bush, and he would run right past me, then abruptly stop and sniff the air. He would catch my scent and make a beeline right to the spot where I was. I might have been a sweaty mess, but I guess I smelled pretty good to him.

* * *

Later that year at a vet appointment, I told Dr. Rice that I was going to take Gabriel to the Crisis Nursery's Christmas party. He said, "Are you nuts, a Weimaraner? Pam, he couldn't be in a crowd like that. With all those kids … are you sure? Weims can be a bit overzealous."

"Oh, I'm taking him!"

I was pleased to report to Dr. Rice that Gabriel had done so well, he was asked to come back and visit the children again. I think Dr. Rice thought I was exaggerating, but he learned otherwise. He said recently, "When you told me that you were going to have Gabriel registered as a therapy dog to work with kids, I thought you were nuts. I was not an early endorser of Gabriel's chosen career because, in my experience, Weimaraners are just a little too hyper for that kind of thing. But as I got to know him, he was the best Weim I'd ever seen. He was calm and easygoing, and he just loved kids."

Then we had a good laugh when I reminded him, "Remember the time when we gave him the rabies vaccine?"

There were some indications that Gabriel might make a good therapy dog, but it wasn't like he had a therapy dog neon sign flashing above his head. I do believe that I played a part in his success because we worked so well as a team. He would do anything for me. I soon noticed something I now believe to be true of all therapy teams: the bond between Gabe and me deepened incredibly once we began working as a therapy team. I'd always had a great bond with Gabe, but the minute we started working as a therapy team, it grew to a level words just can't explain. You can only understand it if you do it. Something about the energy exchange of working together to do something meaningful deepens that bond beyond anything you can imagine.

* * *

In the early stages of the organization, Gabriel always wore a bandana when we were working. I came up with the idea because I needed a way to let him know it was time to go to work, something he could wear every time he visited the children. The bandana worked. He was so focused and thoughtful when wearing it. Yet, he somehow knew he could be a regular dog when he wasn't wearing the bandana. Over time, we moved to a formal therapy vest, much like the ones service dogs wear.

It becomes their uniform, and the dogs connect the vest with working.

I always thought if Gabriel was in the back of my SUV on Sunday morning on the way to the dog park, the caption could have read: "The village idiot goes to the dog park," as he would pant and spin with anticipation of a long game of fetch. Yet the following Monday morning, he'd be in the same SUV with his vest on, going to visit the kids, and the caption might read: "Serious therapy dog, Gabriel, on his way to work." Amazing.

* * *

One instance of hyper Gabe at the dog park is etched in my memory. He was about two years old, and Mike was launching the ball for him to fetch. Gabriel would never end the game on purpose. It seemed as if he might go until he passed out, so it was up to us to monitor when he'd had enough. After about twenty returns by Gabriel, the tennis ball had become a slimy, frothy mess. To make matters worse, Gabriel was foaming at the mouth from all the excitement. We made him take a break and led him over to the water station. All the people were laughing at this frothing, panting dog who looked like he was smiling from ear to ear.

The water station consisted of big pails of water situated on a pile of rocks. Thankfully, no mud. We looked over, and there was huge Gabriel, trying to get into the pail of water — not just take a drink, but actually get *into* the pail. Realizing he wasn't going to succeed, he took a long drink, leaving his foam and drool behind. Done and happy, his tongue was hanging out the side of his mouth. It was a lovely sight. At that point, I was pretty much pretending I didn't know this possessed creature. All the other dogs were walking around calmly, but no, not Gabe. He looked like an escapee from a mental institution.

After a few minutes, I noticed a lady looking intently at him. I casually looked around, like he was *not* my dog. She walked toward us and asked, "Are you Gabriel?" I was absolutely cringing. Yes, this Cujolike creature was mine. She came over and seemed to ask him directly, "Are you Gabriel?"

He looked at her as if to say, "Yeah, I'm Gabriel! Wanna throw my ball?"

I was still cringing, but I said, "Yes, that's Gabriel."

She was suddenly very animated, saying loudly, "I've met him!

I've met him!"

I said dryly, "Oh, that's nice. Where did you meet him?"

"Oh, it was this black-tie affair, and Gabriel was there in a tuxedo!"

"Well, then you must have met me, too, because I was there with him, as we always travel together."

"No," she shook her head, "I don't think I've ever met you. But I definitely met Gabriel." She had no recollection of me, but she was so excited that she'd met Gabriel at a fundraising event. At that moment, he was still panting and drooling everywhere. After all, he was a real dog, having fun and being crazy like a typical Weimaraner. That was probably the first time Gabe was recognized in public, which I would have preferred to have had occur in another venue when he was clean and collected, not in the midst of the possessed, seemingly rabid frenzy that day. But that didn't faze her in the least; she was just so thrilled to see him again.

* * *

Eventually, it wasn't just Gabriel, but Gabriel's Angels that became recognizable. One day I was wearing a Gabriel's Angels shirt when I went into Starbucks, and the barista asked, "Do you work for Gabriel's Angels?"

Hmmm ... how should you answer that one, Pam? "Sort of. I'm Gabriel's mom."

"Oh, my God, Gabriel's mom!" she cried. She turned to her co-worker and loudly repeated, "That's Gabriel's mom!" The coworker had no idea what Gabriel's Angels was, nor who Gabriel was. I just smiled and waited for my latte. As she prepared my coffee, she said proudly, "Oh, I read about Gabriel and all his work with the kids..." It was a repeat of the incident with the lady at the dog park; at that moment, I felt like I'd lost my identity. She knew Gabriel, but had no idea who I was.

Nevertheless, I went home that day and told Mike, "People know who we are now! The Starbucks lady noticed my shirt and knew who we were!"

"Nice." Mike says, "You got one." He has always been there to keep me grounded. As it turned out, however, it was many more than one.

GABRIEL'S ANGELS

* * *

Though I had traveled enough during my corporate life to carry me for quite a while, I did drive up to northern Arizona with my sister a few years back. She was visiting from Florida, and I wanted to show her the beautiful town of Sedona and its famed red rocks. We were there for just a few days and stayed in an obscure little hotel in the downtown area. Aware how important branding and marketing always are, I'd had black and white magnetic pawprints with the Gabriel's Angels logo and information installed on the side of my Tahoe.

While we were at breakfast one morning, I received a text message from a friend: "Are you in Sedona?"

What, are they following me? I thought. *Can't I do anything at all in my private life without someone knowing about it?* Well, no one was following me. My friend had received a phone call from some European relatives who were visiting Sedona before they made their way down to Phoenix. They remembered her talking about Gabriel's Angels, and they had parked right next to my Tahoe. Excited, they called to tell her about the big American car with the Gabriel's Angels pawprints.

It's times like those that keep this work so rich and beautiful. I don't ever want to forget the first visit. I don't ever want to forget the first time someone said, "Oh, I know Gabriel's Angels!" Today it happens quite often, but I still marvel at the fact that people have heard of us and the important work we are doing. I never realized until after he passed away how many people Gabriel touched. There were so many, many cards, all saying things like, "I remember when I met Gabe. I met him here. You brought him there."

* * *

When Gabriel was about four years old, we had a commitment to visit the Crisis Nursery on a Saturday for a big family festival for the preschool children and their parents. The police would be doing fingerprinting, and the fire department was going to be there with their big red truck. It was going to be a fun event, and they asked me if I would bring Gabriel so the parents could meet him, too. I was happy to do so.

When we arrived, I had a large bag with literature and Gabriel in tow. We went out to the playground — the very same playground he visited for his entire career, the playground that was *his* playground.

We were heading out the door when I felt him pull back, stopping in the door well, just shaking. I thought he might be having a seizure, it was so severe.

I had no idea what happening. "Gabriel," I said, "There are people, and there are the kids. This is what you do best." But he wouldn't look up and he was still shaking violently. For one quick second, I did see him glance up, so I followed his line of sight to see what he was looking at. The nursery had set up a bouncy for the kids in the play area. On the top of the bouncy was a replica of Shamu, the Killer Whale. My poor Gabriel was convinced it was real, and Shamu was after him. Gabriel wanted out, and he wanted out NOW. I was so worried for him — and quite embarrassed at the same time.

He was so upset that I couldn't reason with him. I couldn't tell him it was okay, because Shamu the Killer Whale was going to kill *him*. In his dog mind, it was fight or flight, so he flew! In his effort to get away from Shamu, Gabe pulled me to my knees and my literature went flying everywhere. I could hear the parents murmuring, "Oh, *that's* Gabriel, the therapy dog?"

One of the staff members finally opened the side door to allow Gabriel and me to enter the building, far out of Shamu's sight. He was still trembling, and I could not get him to calm down. Finally, I said his name. "GABRIEL! It's okay. You're okay. We are inside now." We stayed in the lobby for quite some time, as he frantically panted and panted. I told the staff person, "I think we need to go."

She was very understanding, "No problem. We hope Gabriel will be okay."

And so we were back home within thirty minutes of departing. By now, Gabe had stopped panting and was completely calm. Mike looked at me and asked, "Didn't you just leave?" I told him the story about big, scary Shamu, and we had a laugh.

Later the same day, Gabriel was out in our backyard; I was still watching him because of his ordeal. I felt so sorry I had put him in that situation and I knew he was still a bit freaked out. As I watched him wander around, he looked up and began shaking violently again. I screamed to Mike, "I told you it was a seizure! Something is wrong!!"

Mike came running out while Gabe continued to shake. Suddenly Gabriel glanced up for a moment, just as he had at the nursery. So again,

I followed the line to see where he was looking. Our next door neighbor's yard is separated from ours by a typical nine-foot cement wall, quite common in the Phoenix area. Normally, it was benignly bland. That day, however, was their daughter's fifth birthday, and the neighbors had rented a *bouncy* for her birthday party. What are the chances?

Not only had this poor dog had a close encounter with Shamu, but now he was facing a very scary dragon. Shamu … dragon … it was all the same to Gabriel. He again went into fight or flight, and my dog was no fighter. It was a bad day for Gabriel, and it was six months before he could look up again without trembling. Time heals many things, and Gabriel fully recovered and was eventually even able to attend a neighborhood event that had a few "headless" bouncies.

* * *

The things poor Gabe endured. One August, Gabriel and I were invited to speak to a very high-level Soroptimist club in Downtown Phoenix. The event took place at the Arizona Club, which is on the thirty-eighth floor of the Chase Building, one of the tallest buildings in the city. The speaker coordinator had asked me to talk to their club about our pet therapy program and told me they wanted to meet Gabriel. It worked out well because later that afternoon, I needed to attend a trade show with Gabriel, also in Downtown Phoenix. Rarely do things work out so well when scheduling appearances. It felt like a lucky day.

Gabriel and I arrived in the parking garage with plenty of time to spare. We walked into the elevator, and Gabriel looked up at me, a bit perplexed, because no matter how often we did it, he didn't seem to understand the concept of getting into a small room that moved vertically. To make matters worse, this particular elevator was an express, so it moved a bit faster than usual. As the doors closed and we began to ascend, I looked down at Gabriel who was sprawled out on all fours, like GI Joe. The other people in the elevator laughed as they asked, "Is he okay?"

"Yes, he's fine. He just doesn't understand the concept of the elevator."

The elevator stopped and we exited to a very posh restaurant, where all the exterior walls are floor-to-ceiling glass that offer an amazing view of the entire city. Gabriel immediately walked over to the glass walls and his ears went up — it was as if he was saying, "Ooohhhhh, that's how these elevator things work!" As far as he was concerned, we were at the top of the world.

As requested, I spoke to the women judges and attorneys in atten-dance about Gabriel's Angels and our work to intervene in the cycle of violence. Gabriel was the consummate gentleman. I remember it as one of the times I was most proud of him. I finished speaking and thought, *Perfect. My car is in the covered parking garage, and I need to be about four blocks away in a half-hour or so.* I was wearing moderate heels, so I decided I'd be comfortable enough to walk these few blocks.

You must understand, Downtown was a bit intimidating to me be-cause I was unfamiliar with the layout. Whenever I had a meeting or event in Downtown Phoenix, I felt I was being punished in some way. *What did I do wrong?* and *I'm sure I'll get lost* were my usual reactions, probably because of all the one-way streets. But today, I had looked at a map and knew where I was going! I would just head up three blocks and over one, and Gabe and I would be right where we needed to be. So off we went.

It was August in Phoenix, which translates to H-O-T, but I was sure we'd be okay because we didn't have far to go. Just two blocks into our walk, I felt like a very bad doggie mom, because there was poor Gabriel, dancing on the sidewalk like a prancing horse. Of course! I had on mod-erately high heels, but he was in bare paws! I looked around frantically for some grass for him to stand on. But this was Downtown Phoenix — concrete everywhere. I glanced around again and saw St. Mary's Ba-silica, so we ran over there and I led him to some shade on the grass. I sensed that Gabe was starting to panic. Meanwhile, I was thinking, *I've got two blocks to the Phoenix Convention Center, and it's two blocks back to the parking garage.* I was stuck right in the middle, with Gabriel's doggie boots conveniently in the car.

I had no choice but to go for it. Gabriel and I began running through Downtown. Running. In Phoenix. In August. Gabe in his bare paws and I in my moderately high heels ran as fast as we could. Every time I saw any shade, I stopped for him. But each time we stopped, it was still hot. Finally we saw the Civic Center, our oasis in the desert! By now my face was streaming sweat, my neatly pressed suit was a rumpled mess, and Gabriel was panting hard. We came running up to the Convention Center in all of our glory. To the people in line registering, we must have looked like we'd just been dropped from a spaceship.

Concerned, they asked, "Is your dog okay?"

"Yes," I panted. "It's ... just ... that we had ... to run ... over here." I didn't need to tell them the whole story. They brought Gabriel some water. I'm not sure that I was ever offered a bottle of water, but at least Gabe got a drink so he could cool down.

Lesson learned. I never again went anywhere without booties for Gabriel in the summer. I was caught unprepared this time and pledged it would never happen again.

After we cooled off, we mingled with the attendees at the trade show, and everything went fine. It was five o'clock, and nearly one hundred and ten degrees outside. The pavement was probably closer to one hundred forty degrees. I realized, *I'm kind of stuck here, because my car is four blocks away, and no way am I walking back with Gabriel.*

A lady I'd met at the event offered to help. She told me, "My husband is driving to the front of the building to pick up some of my supplies, so he can take you and Gabriel to the parking garage. We have a duel truck, so you and Gabriel can sit in the back."

Perfect, I thought.

"But," she said, "we have to wait outside, because I told my husband I'd flag him down as he drives around."

That was fine. At least we were going to get a ride. I offered to help her carry some things out to the curb, so I asked the head of the Promotional Products Association and a few of her friends to watch Gabe. They were delighted to be asked. Said at least five women in unison, "Of course we'll watch him!"

Reassured that Gabriel was in good hands, I made another trip outside to help carry some boxes. As we made our way to the curb, my new friend saw her husband in his little truck. She pointed him out, and we waved our hands all over the place. He drove right past us.

She said, "I guess he didn't see us."

He made another trip around the block, and we were waving like maniacs now, shouting, "Over here! Over here!" Still, he didn't see us. Well, I wasn't going to stand around trying to help her flag down her confused husband while my dog was inside with the ladies. She called him on his cell phone, but he didn't answer. He was apparently lost, and at this point, I didn't know what else to do.

I looked around and noticed this guy on a bicycle, pulling behind him what appeared to be a bench on wheels. The Arizona Diamondbacks baseball team had a game that night at their Downtown stadium, and these bicycle rickshaws were a common sight on game nights, driving people back and forth from parking lots to the field. I yelled at the driver, "STOP!" Again, I was sweating profusely and looked a fright.

He pulled over next to me and asked, "Are you okay?"

"I'm fine. But I need to know if you will take me to the Chase Bank tower?"

"Sure, I can do that," he said agreeably.

"There's only one catch."

He asked, "What's that?"

"Will you also take my dog?"

He smiled and said, "I love dogs!"

I said, "Great. Stay right here." So I went running back into the Civic Center, looking everywhere for Gabriel. I didn't see him anywhere. Finally, over in the corner, there was now a cluster of some twenty women, all gathered around Gabriel petting him. He was just soaking up the attention while they smiled and laughed and talked. Finally, though, he caught my eye, and I motioned to him to come. He came over to me at once. We headed toward the door. Over my shoulder, I called, "Thank you, ladies, for watching him for me!"

I led Gabriel over to the rickshaw and said, "You can do this."

He just looked at me, as if to say, "OK!"

On seeing Gabe, the rickshaw driver said, "That's a big dog!" Now you must understand, this vehicle was a little bench with a little back. Nothing elaborate like those horse-drawn carriages you see in New York City. This was a bicycle pulling a cart behind it — *very* basic.

I told Gabriel again, "You can do this," and he was already standing on the foot plate, like, "Let's go!" I hoisted him up so he was sitting up in the rickshaw like a person. I climbed in next to him, and we were sitting there like a couple. Lovely. The driver was just looking at me, a bit unsure. "He can do this," I said.

"Seems so," he agreed. Gabriel leaned into me, and I wrapped my arms around him. The rickshaw guy took off like we'd been shot out of a cannon! He flew down First Avenue on the sidewalk. Gabriel's ears were flapping in the wind, hitting me in the face. Then the driver took a left-hand turn, and we flew off the sidewalk, down a ramp, across the intersection, and back onto the sidewalk. By now, cars were stopping to watch the giant gray dog flying through Downtown Phoenix behind a bicycle. I was holding onto him for dear life. Drivers and passengers rolled their windows down, extended their arms, and pointed at us every step of the way. But the rickshaw driver was not slowing down for anything. For me, it was scary and fun at the same time. For Gabriel, it was just fun. Finally we arrived at parking garage elevator bank, in one piece.

I breathed a huge sigh, "You are a godsend!"

The driver smiled, "That's the first time I ever took a dog anywhere!"

"What do I owe you?" I asked him.

"Well, for you … for a human … it's twenty dollars," he said. "But I don't know what to charge for the dog."

I said, "Here's forty dollars, because you got us here in one piece." I was happy to depart with that cash. Gabriel and I took the elevator up, and I got him into the back of the car. As I was driving home, I looked in the rearview mirror, and he was standing up with a look on his face like, "That was so much fun! Can we do it again?"

Imagine all the people stopping in the street on the way to the ballpark to see this huge dog in the rickshaw. He pretty much just leaned on me, and we did it. That was one of the great things about Gabriel. If I told him it was okay, he knew it was okay. We had a trusting bond, and he trusted me enough to take that ride.

CHAPTER EIGHT

The Children

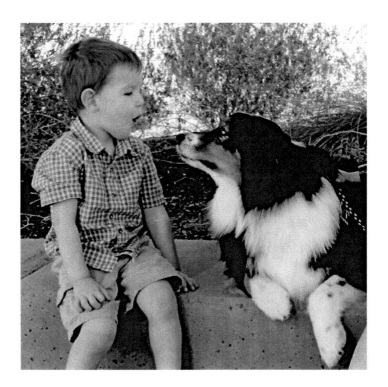

The children at the Crisis Nursery and places like it are not there by choice. As often as not, their behavior would be totally unacceptable in the real world. But the thing I've come to understand is that their behavior is the reason they're still alive. They didn't have safe, comfortable homes with families who loved them, so they learned how to protect themselves and how to stop someone from hitting them. They may seem aggressive and ill-mannered, but that's the reason they're still here. When you understand that, you see how the dogs can help break through and reach these children in a way that even the best-intentioned adult humans simply cannot.

However, not every child is immediately accepting of the therapy dogs. These children don't have anyone advocating for them, so they become very desensitized. Early on, one little boy really didn't seem to care for Gabriel at all. As our visit progressed, I was more than a little shocked to hear him say, "My dad shot my dog." In his reality, though, it was just another violent episode among many in his short life. And he had made the self-protective decision that he would never love another dog, because someone might hurt it. He never wanted to feel that kind of loss again. Now I understood why he did not like Gabriel. This young boy had built a wall to shield himself from future disappointments.

* * *

Even the children who did immediately bond with Gabriel didn't necessarily trust him. That's why trust is one of the most important traits we work to develop in these kids. Early in his career at Crisis Nursery, Gabe met a little girl who was about five years old. We arrived during nap time, and she was sound asleep. She woke before the other kids, rubbed her eyes, and said, "Hi, big gray dog."

I asked, "What's your name?"

"My name is Tatiana."

"Well, this is Gabriel." Tatiana began to pet Gabe's soft fur. As the other kids woke up, she took Gabriel's leash and began introducing him to all the kids. She completely took over. It was so sweet.

One at a time, Tatiana introduced Gabe to each of the children, "Hi, this is Gabriel. You can pet him. He's my friend." Then to the next kid, "This is Gabriel. You can pet him." This went on for about an hour. When it was time for Gabe and me to leave, all the children hugged Gabriel and said goodbye. Tatiana asked me when he was coming back.

I said, "We will be back next week, Tatiana."

She said a soft, "Hmmm," and went to the kitchen where the children were gathering for a snack. Children who are victims of abuse and neglect have learned to distrust adults in order to shield themselves from disappointment. The next week, Gabe and I returned, as promised. Tatiana came running up to us, screaming, "Gabriel, you came back, you came back!!

THE CHILDREN

Hey everybody, Gabriel came back!!" I didn't understand why she was so surprised to see Gabriel, as I had told her we'd be coming back next week.

A staff member pulled me aside and explained that after our previous visit, Tatiana had told all the children, "He's not coming back, so don't expect him to. He won't keep his promise to come back." At such a tender age, Tatiana was shielding herself from disappointment by expecting that Gabriel would not return. She'd already had so many disappointments in her young life that she refused to put her trust in anyone or anything, Gabriel included.

Well, we kept coming back, and every week Tatiana was amazed! She formed a strong attachment to him, and eventually learned to trust that he would continue to keep his word. Her relationship with Gabriel was probably the first healthy attachment she had formed. Instilling trust in children who were victims of abuse and neglect was one of Gabe's greatest talents.

Trust is the foundation for everything because it leads to behavioral development in other areas. One of the hardest things to gauge is tolerance. How can you really tell if a six-, seven-, eight-, nine-, or ten-year-old kid is becoming more tolerant? We measure tolerance as a core behavior because we know it intervenes in the cycle of violence. People who have learned these behaviors — respect, compassion, empathy, trust, affiliation, tolerance, and self-esteem — aren't in the cycle of violence. Whether they were fortunate enough to never have been a part of the cycle, or they had an intervening experience like pet therapy, people who live these traits simply are not violent.

* * *

Sometimes, the dogs' most important function is just being there to offer comfort and companionship. A four-year-old boy, Devon, was living at the Crisis Nursery. During one of our visits, he wasn't with the other children, so I asked, "Where's Devon?"

The staff told me, "Well, he had a rather rough morning, so we thought it would be best if we didn't subject Gabriel to his antics." They were just being protective of Gabriel. As we were getting ready to leave, we saw Devon and one of the teachers coming down the hall. Devon's eyes were swollen shut from crying, his lips were still quivering, and he couldn't catch his breath.

I looked at him and asked, "Hey, Devon, do you want to see Gabriel?"

"Oh-oh-oh-kay-ay," he said, starting to cry again. I walked Gabriel over to him, and he put his arms around Gabriel's neck. And there they went (with me behind, holding onto the leash) walking down the hall together. It was so precious. After about ten minutes with Gabriel, Devon looked much calmer and happier. I think Gabriel's "thereness," or perhaps better said, his constantly soothing presence during his visits with the children, was the source of his ability to calm them down. I sensed that just by being there, Gabriel made the children feel less lonely, less afraid, and less anxious.

Later that day, I was working in my home office and I received a call from the nursery. "We just wanted to thank you."

That was unexpected. "What for?" I asked.

"Well, because of you, Devon had a great rest of the day."

I told them, "Don't thank me. Thank the gray dog laying next to me."

Clearly, there's more happening through our visits than we will ever know. Having a pet can reduce heart rate and calm us down — but it also makes us more social. Isolated people can benefit from taking their dog for a walk; it gets them out and gives them the opportunity to become better socialized. There are many other health benefits. Take loneliness. You don't have to take your pet outside — sometimes a pet just gives you someone to talk to. I remember being in the den with Gabriel one time when I told him, "I love you." Mike yelled from another room, "I love you, too." I was thinking, *I wasn't talking to you!* But I yelled back, "Thank you!"

* * *

Gabe wasn't the only therapy dog in the family. My Rhodesian Ridgeback, Noah (who has since retired), and I made regular visits to the teenage boys in a group home. A boy named Carlos was normally very active with Noah and loved to hang out with us. One day when we arrived, Carlos — sixteen at the time — was sitting in a lawn chair outside. A staff counselor sat facing him, and Carlos looked like he had lost his best friend. He wouldn't look up; he seemed sullen and very depressed. As I pulled into the parking lot, the other boys helped me get Noah out of the car. I didn't go over to where Carlos was sitting because

I could see that something heavy duty was going on.

About half-an-hour into our visit, I noticed that the counselor had left, but Carlos was still sitting there. So I said, "Hey, Carlos. Come over here." He didn't really respond, so I continued, "Noah wants to see you. He came all the way from Ahwatukee ... you need to come see Noah." He begrudgingly got up, and I said, "You know Carlos, I'm really glad you came over, because Noah could really use a walk. Why don't you take him to that field over there? He would like to share some time with you, just the two of you."

Carlos took the leash, and it was the saddest sight ... two little souls walking away. When they were about thirty yards away, Carlos fell to his knees and began hugging Noah. Noah gently wagged his tail, as if he was giving Carlos reassurance. I didn't see Carlos crying, but he continued to hug Noah. I pointed this out to one of the counselors, who said, "Wow, that's pretty neat."

Carlos walked Noah around a little more and came back after about ten minutes. He had a little smile on his face, so I asked him, "How are you doing?"

He looked at me and said, "Noah's my best friend."

"Well, I'm really glad you came over to see him, because you made Noah's day, too." I hadn't asked, so I still didn't know what was going on — but with these kids, with teenagers, you never know. It could be something small, or it could be a really big deal. Carlos stayed with us the rest of the time, and when the boys all went in to dinner, I asked the counselor who had been sitting with Carlos when we arrived, "What's going on with him?"

He told me that Carlos' mom had decided she didn't want to see him anymore. She had relinquished her guardianship of him, and she wasn't going to visit him any longer. After receiving this news, he had been despondent all day. Since ten o'clock that morning, he hadn't spoken to anyone, hadn't looked at anyone, hadn't done anything. And now he'd just gone skipping into the house to eat dinner. "It shows the power of having these dogs come visit here," the counselor said. "The other counselors and I couldn't reach Carlos, but Noah — just being Noah and without knowing anything — brought him out of his shell."

I don't know that Carlos wouldn't have come out of his despair otherwise, but I do know that he came out of it rather quickly because of

Noah. I was proud that Noah could do that for him. It was just a really special time. We were in exactly the right place at the right time.

Many children we deal with have built hard shells around themselves, shells that protect them from the outside world. I have been privileged to witness the unconditional love of therapy dogs cracking fissures in the shells to reach those children. When there's love, there's hope, and when there's hope, anything is possible.

Without knowing the full story, it may be tempting to think, *Carlos' parents are just awful.* But the thing I've learned along the way is that I don't know their story. I don't know what Carlos did or didn't do. I don't know how long the situation has been going on.

In instances when I have been onsite and a parent has visited, I held no judgment. I don't know why that mother who came to visit her boys at the Crisis Nursery was loud or dirty or what many people would consider unpresentable. I don't know her story, but I do know that her kids were safe. Maybe she simply had the sense to put her kids in the Crisis Nursery so she could go figure out what to do with her life. In this work, you quickly learn that you can't make assumptions.

* * *

When teenage boys arrive at the agency I used to visit with Noah, they enter at Phase 1, which means they have no privileges until they prove they are responsible. Once they adhere to the rules and exhibit good behavior, they can move to the next phase. After they hit Phase 4, I generally don't see them anymore, because they are moved to an agency with less oversight as they prepare to enter the adult world. They usually go to one of the homes in town where they attend a regular high school and get a part-time job. They may even go home.

Sometimes, when Noah and I were visiting the boys, I'd ask, "What phase are you this week?"

One boy answered, "Two."

"Wait," I said. "You were Phase 3 last week. You must have had a bad week."

"You don't want to know about it."

Fair enough. I probably didn't want to know.

But one time, I received a specific answer, "I got a lower phase because I disrespected a staff member."

"Now isn't that interesting, that you would choose to disrespect a staff member?"

"Nah-ah," he responded. "It wasn't my fault. The staff member made me angry, so I disrespected him."

I repeated, "Isn't that just so interesting that you would choose to disrespect him?" I have always been really big on personal responsibility, and so is the staff at this group home. Yet, it's fairly typical for youth not to take responsibility. It's our job to teach them to not play the victim role. By working with Noah, the boys and I developed a trusting relationship, and they felt they could be honest with me.

* * *

Many of the kids we work with are Hispanic and don't speak English fluently. When the English-speaking children said, "Gabriel, sit. Gabriel, stay," he obliged. But when the Hispanic children would say: "Gabriel, siéntate. Gabriel, quieto," poor Gabriel would cock his head and look at them, trying to understand what they wanted from him.

I had taught Gabriel hand commands when he was a puppy. I suppose it's akin to sign language for dogs. The command of raising my hand into an UP position from the elbow meant "Sit." So I would stand behind the kids. They'd be facing Gabe so they couldn't see me, and they would say "Gabriel, siéntate. Siéntate!" Standing behind them, I raised my hand, and he sat. The children were shocked. They yelled, "Miss Pam, Miss Pam, Gabriel knows Spanish!" They were so excited and happy.

My English-speaking kids would say, "Gabriel, down." And the Spanish-speaking kids would say, "Gabriel, abajo. Abajo!" The hand command for DOWN is to put your hand straight up in the air. Gabriel knew this one well. So when the children said, "Gabriel, abajo!" I'd stick my arm in the air, and sure enough, he went down. So again, the kids were delighted. "Miss Pam, Miss Pam, Gabriel knows Spanish!" Seeing the joy on their faces, I didn't have the heart to tell them that it was really my signs he was reading.

I was home with Gabe about a week later, and he was staring intently at the doggie cookie jar on the counter. I said, "Gabriel, sientate." He promptly sat. I just looked at him. So then I said, "Abajo?" and he laid down. Nah, the dog could not possibly have learned Spanish, so I figured I'd really challenge him. "Dame tu mano," I said, and he gave me his paw. Gabe had learned Spanish from those kids. Further proof that absolutely anything was possible.

Later that year, Gabriel was a guest on one of the local Spanish television stations. I remember Patricio Benito was speaking Spanish about a hundred miles an hour, but somewhere in there he said, "Sientate," and Gabriel sat. Patricio kept talking, blah-blah-blah in Spanish, and then, "Dame tu mano," and Gabriel put out his paw. The capacity for Gabriel to learn Spanish astonished me. Initially he associated the hand signal with the Spanish word, but eventually the word itself was good enough. My dog was tri-lingual! English, Spanish, and sign language.

Spanish phrases Gabriel knew

Siéntate — Sit.

Quieto — Stay.

Abajo — Down.

Levantarse — Get up.

Dame tu mano — Give me your hand.

Ven aquí — Come here.

Vámanos — Let's go.

Representatives from Gabriel's Angels often speak to groups of kids, like a Boy Scout troop or a school, and afterward the scout leaders or teachers have the kids send thank-you notes. Almost invariably, their favorite thing about Gabriel was that he knew three languages. "Miss Pam, Gabriel knows English, Spanish, and sign language. That was my most favorite thing!"

Children need to experience healthy power. So often, the children we work with feel powerless because the only power they see is unhealthy violence from the adults in their lives. When you let a ten-year-old walk a dog, and allow him to instruct, "Gabriel, sit. Gabriel, stay. Gabriel, come," that's power, but it's a positive, healthy power. It's not a domineering, controlling power over an animal. When a five-year-old gives the dog a treat, and all the kids start high-fiving each other because they're so excited that the dog accepted the treat, that's something very special to see.

* * *

Eventually the kids at the Crisis Nursery graduate and move on from pre-school to kindergarten. Every year, Gabriel was invited to the pre-school graduation. He would sponsor one child's cap and gown, so he got the invitation. I only went because Gabe didn't drive. And even though they saw him every week, Gabriel was like a rock star with these kids. Gabriel would arrive, and you could hear the children yelling, "Gabriel's here! Gabriel's here!" It was like a celebrity had entered the building.

When we arrived for the graduations, I was always very careful to keep Gabe hidden, because if they knew he was there, no one would be able to focus on the ceremony. There would be plenty of time to mix and mingle after the diplomas had been handed out. I stood with all the adults behind a circular half wall in the small room so the children couldn't see Gabe as they marched in. The kids were to sit on their little chairs in the middle of the room.

The program began, but Gabe was well hidden. Perfect! As you might expect, a lot of the kids were fidgeting during the ceremony; some were looking around at their parents and whoever else was there. Right in the middle of the ceremony, little Tabitha saw me and yelled out, "Hey everybody, there's the lady that brings the dog!" Everybody laughed, and I just shrugged, "Sorry."

The next year at graduation, I was trying to hide Gabriel during the handing out of the diplomas, but he decided he was very interested in watching. No longer satisfied to sit quietly, Gabriel put his paws up on the half wall so he could see the ceremony. Before I could get him back down, little Devon yelled, "Hey, everybody, there's Gabriel!"

* * *

One cute little girl named Gabrielle — Gabby for short — took a real liking to Gabe. She was just in love with him. She would light up when she saw him and gently hang on his neck. As Gabriel walked around the nursery, Gabby would put her arm around his neck and walk with him. Though she was at the Crisis Nursery, Gabby hadn't been removed from her family. She was part of a daycare program for area residents, so I saw her mother pick her up a number of times. One day her mom came over and said, "Oh, you must be Gabriel. All Gabby talks about is Gabriel, Gabriel, Gabriel."

GABRIEL'S ANGELS

Gabby started attending the Crisis Nursery pre-school when she was about a year old. Because of a hearing impairment, she was late to develop speech. "She'd say one word sentences," says Lissa, her mom. "Things like 'Mommy' and 'Daddy.' One day, she came home saying 'Doggie. Doggie. Doggie.' We later learned from her teacher that Gabriel had begun visiting the nursery.

"Gabby had an immediate bond with Gabriel," Lissa explains. "Because their names are so similar, she felt she had a special connection to him, and he always cheered her up. The staff told me she would never take a nap on the days Gabriel visited, because she didn't want to miss out on any time with him." As a result of her hearing and speech challenges, Gabby always felt a little different. Watching Gabriel recuperate from his first surgery and come bounding back to work at the nursery made her feel like she could be better, too.

"Gabriel was always a big part of everything she did," Lissa says. "One time, Gabriel was at the nursery. Although she'd always been a bit afraid of heights, Gabby got up on the monkey bars that day and made it all the way across, just to show Gabriel that she could do it. He gave her the courage and confidence to try something new because he was there watching and supporting her."

Gabrielle graduated some time ago and is now in grammar school where she's doing very well. In May 2010, she came home from school crying because she'd heard from a classmate that a dog named Gabriel had died. The little boy told her about an article in The Arizona Republic titled "Gabriel Gets His Wings: Beloved Therapy Dog Dies of Cancer." Gabby went home that day sobbing, "Mommy, Mommy, Gabriel died. I heard about it at school."

Lissa called to tell me how sorry they were, and how sad Gabby was that Gabriel wasn't here anymore. Gabby had said to Lissa, "He has to be in heaven now, Mom, because he was one of the angels." Gabby is eight now, but her mom tells me she still has photos of herself with me and Gabe. She's so proud of them — she always shows them to anyone new she meets. Her mom reminded me that I had a special nickname for her, Gabby Gabs-a-Lot, because that kid is always talking.

"I'm so grateful for the work that Gabriel's Angels does," Lissa says. "They really help these kids in a very special way. They give them hope and support and encouragement. It's always interesting to me to hear people in the community talk about Gabriel's Angels, because I know from the inside what an amazing job they do."

After Gabe passed, I sent Gabby a little care package with a small stuffed Weimaraner, a Gabriel's Angels backpack, Gabriel's Memorial Trading Card, and short note from me about how much Gabriel loved her. I can't help but believe this illustrates the fact that Gabriel touched the children he worked with in ways I will never know.

Once they leave the agency providing the care, we have no further contact. It meant a lot when Lissa called after hearing of Gabe's death to tell me how much Gabby still loved him. She was only five years old when she left the preschool program, but she'd never forgotten him. My unique relationship with Gabby and her mom is a special side blessing of this work.

* * *

One interesting thing is that we really don't know how much the therapy dog takes in, or how this work ultimately affects the dog's health. Do they feel the angst and unsettledness of the children? Gabriel worked with more kids than any other therapy dog to date. He probably reached about 10,000 kids, personally. That's a lot of kids.

I have no way of knowing how many children's lives were changed forever, but I do know that they all benefited from this therapy dog's unconditional love. I also know there is a lot more going on than we can see on the surface. Although most of the kids eventually move on and I don't know what happens next in their lives, I do have two boys from the group home Noah and I used to visit, now in their early twenties, who stay in touch with me. It's nice that they let me know how they're doing.

Ernest is one of the boys who keeps in touch. He's twenty-three now, living in Prescott Valley, Arizona, where his family has always lived, even while he was down in Phoenix at the boys' home. Ernest was one of the few kids who got to meet all three of my dogs: Gabriel, Noah, and Jack. "The biggest thing I think I got from working with Gabriel," Ernest explains, "was confidence to do important things. Taking care of him made me feel like I could do anything."

CHAPTER NINE

Gabriel Adjusts to Canine Siblings

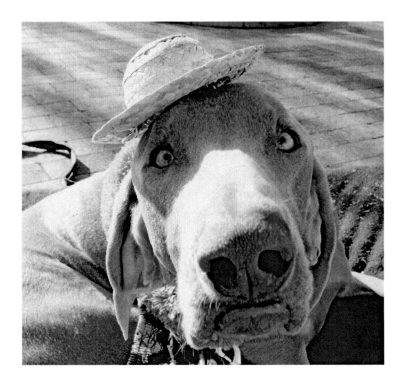

When Gabriel joined our family, he was entering a household already oc-
cupied by two four-legged children: our two adult cats. I was concerned
that this exuberant puppy could inadvertently hurt them, as he would
not understand their lack of interest in this "playing" activity. I asked my
dog trainer what to do, and she simply said, "Jessie and Orzo will handle
Gabriel. He has a sweet demeanor and would not hurt them."

"What do you mean?" I was a bit concerned that either she hadn't heard me properly, or she wasn't taking me seriously.

She repeated, "Let the cats handle it." Obviously, I didn't like this answer. The trainer explained, "If you don't let them handle it, they will never have a relationship with Gabriel. Your cats could learn to fear him. This young pup needs to respect that the cats were here first."

I did as she said and didn't intervene, but I closely watched over them all. As Gabriel would run up to the cats, they'd hiss. Sometimes Jessie would run from him, and I would say, "If you don't run, no one can chase you." All of a sudden I thought, *Oh my God, I'm turning into my mother!* When I was ten, she had instructed me not to run from the boys on the playground, using the exact same words.

It was Orzo, the younger cat, who taught Gabriel a very valuable lesson about respect. Orzo was five years old at the time, and he was sitting on a chair in the kitchen one morning. Gabriel came racing around the corner and slid into Orzo's furry belly. Orzo stood up on his hind legs just like a bear, and in the time it took the clock to tick one second, he batted Gabriel across the face about fifty times. Gabriel's eyes were huge. He shook his head and quietly walked away. Well into his adult years, Gabriel had a scar on his nose from that encounter. But from that moment on, the level of respect Gabriel had for the cats was amazing.

Jessie has since passed away, but to this day, Orzo can walk by our dogs with his tail straight up in the air. He will walk underneath Jack, my current Weimaraner, and the tip of his tail will brush across Jack's belly. I always tell people that Gabriel was raised by cats. They had a great relationship.

* * *

Exactly two years to the day that Gabriel came to live with us, another dog joined our family. It was January 1, 2001, when Mike and I adopted a Rhodesian Ridgeback puppy. We thought it was time for Gabriel to have a little brother to play with. We named the new guy Noah.

I had always heard that two dogs are easier than one, and it's absolutely true. They hang out together, like a two-dog pack. I soon learned, however, that three dogs is a part-time job.

Noah came from a family who also raised exotic birds. We chose his breed for more or less the same reasons we had chosen the Weimaraner:

big dog, short coat, no shedding. That's just my preference. Some people like small, long-haired dogs. I like all dogs, but I'm drawn to the big ones. Mike and I both liked that particular style of dog. Noah was the only puppy left in the litter, but we got to meet his mom, dad, and aunt. We were happy to take home this little "Scrappy Doo" lookalike.

As Noah entered our home, Gabriel looked at him like, "He's really cute. When's he leaving?"

Gabriel, who at this point considered himself the ultimate therapy dog, now had this little pup always chasing after him to play. At two years of age, Gabe was never interested in playing with the other dogs at the dog park. He was only interested in fetching the ball, again and again. But as time went on, I saw the bond between Gabriel and Noah strengthen.

Gabriel taught Noah the ropes, like how to run around the yard, which bushes were best to pee on, and how to be on the lookout for coyotes. They grew up together, and Noah became a therapy dog, too. Unlike Gabe, Noah worked with teenage boys. So I had a really interesting dichotomy: Gabriel working with pre-schoolers, while Noah and I visited the teenage boys. This inadvertently helped improve Gabriel's Angels, because it enabled me to get better at indentifying which person, which dog, and which therapy team should work in which arena. Noah retired in 2008 due to arthritic hips.

* * *

In 2005, the daughter of a friend of mine rescued a Weimaraner named Josee. Her timing was a little odd, as the girl was a full-time student at Arizona State University, and the poor dog was spending eight hours a day in a crate while she attended class. Finding Josee a new home seemed the only right thing to do. So my friend called me to ask, "Do you know anyone who might want to adopt a Weimaraner?"

"No, I really don't," I was quick to answer. But I thought about it and remembered hearing of a lady who might be interested. "Well, maybe. Let me take a look at little Josee."

I went to meet her. Standing there was this perfect little dog, a petite Weimaraner. I sat with her, petted her, and loved on her — and before you know it, she was in *my* car. I was taking her home for a "play date" so we could see if it would work out. We were just going to *see*.

I came home with Josee and put her in the backyard. Mike let Gabriel and Noah out, and they sniffed her, but there was no trouble at all. That first night, they all got along. No problems of any kind. Josee seemed to fit in pretty well with our family. This was June 2005, and I now had three dogs and two cats.

Not surprisingly, it turned out that Josee had not been well socialized; we first noticed the signs at the dog park. A few times, she would chase dogs that obviously did not want to play, insisting that they engage with her anyway. She either hadn't learned to read other dogs very well, or simply didn't care to.

November came, and Mike had to go down to Rocky Point, Mexico, for a couple days on a work trip. I had taken Josee to the boys' group home so she could get some training to become a therapy dog. She was very bright, and I thought she would be good with pre-teens. Josee was a therapy puppy in training; working with the boys helped sharpen her basic skills. I'd had her with me that whole day, and she was obviously bonding with me. When we arrived home, Gabriel and Noah were quite happy to see me. As I removed Josee's work vest, I said, "Hi, guys. I'm just going to put my keys in the office, and then I'll feed you." I turned my back, and all hell broke loose.

I wheeled around to see Josee viciously attacking Gabriel. And I do mean viciously. He was in a defensive position — his body in a circle — just was trying to get away from her, but she was on top of him. I flew out of the office, grabbed her back legs, and pulled her — but I lost my grip, and she went back to attack Gabe again. I was screaming, "Josee, NO!! Josee, NO!!" I pulled her again, and again I lost my grip on her. She seemed unnaturally strong. It was like what they say about people who go crazy, that they can develop superhuman strength. The third time, I remember saying to myself, "You need to be like the Hulk. Don't let her go!" I grabbed her and got her off of Gabe, pushing her up against a wall and yelling, "Josee, Josee, Josee!!"

She looked up at me, shook her head, and suddenly her face cleared, as if she had been in a trance. She was like, "What?"

Then there was Noah, my one-hundred-pound Ridgeback, cowering in the corner with a look on his face like, "Help! What's happening here?" I was fortunate, because most dogs would have had a pack mentality, and they all would have fought. But Noah just stood there like,

GABRIEL ADJUSTS TO CANINE SIBLINGS

"I'm not going in there — she's crazy!"

I looked over, and Gabriel was dripping blood from his ears. He had a large tear under his neck and his eye was swelling shut right in front of me, but I knew he wasn't going to die from his injuries. I was immensely grateful for that, because I was so traumatized at that point that if I'd gotten into the car to take him to the vet, I'm pretty sure we would have crashed. I gated Josee in one of the back rooms without saying a word to her. Mike was away, and I didn't know what else to do, so I huddled with Gabriel in the closet, crying for most of the night.

Up at the crack of dawn, I put Gabriel in the car — I still didn't look at Josee — and I drove him to Dr. Rice's office. They opened at seven thirty, so I parked and waited for the receptionist to open the door. I walked in with Gabriel, crying. Dr. Rice immediately came out and said, "Gabriel, you look like you were tossed out of a pickup truck going fifty miles an hour. What happened?"

"Josee tried to kill Gabe."

Gabriel ended up needing about fifteen stitches around his neck area, and we weren't able to tell until the swelling in his eye went down whether he had any corneal damage. And his ears, those velvety soft ears — we just had to let them heal.

The next day, Mike flew in from Mexico. Now, sometimes with men, you want to wait until they are home and relaxed to tell them something important. In this situation, I didn't have that luxury. Josee was gated up in the back of the house, and Gabriel looked like a prize fighter. Mike called me from the cab, and I said, "OK. You have a choice. I can either tell you what happened now, while you're still in the cab, or you can wait till you get home, but it's not good news so I recommend you choose the first option. I need to know what you want to do, because there won't be any five or ten minutes of chilling out and looking at the mail when you get home."

"Tell me now," he said. So I did.

Mike came in the front door, but he never looked at Josee again. I really don't think he could, because he was so sad for Gabriel. That was his beloved Gabriel, his dog — and she had hurt him in a vicious attack, so he couldn't even look at her. I didn't know what to do. I called a local rescue where I knew the CEO, and I said, "I know you don't take dogs off the street, but please help me."

The next day, I took Josee to the rescue where a behaviorist analyzed her and told me, "This dog is not people aggressive. She's an alpha dog and will always dominate all other dogs in the pack. She can only be in a home without any other pets." She told me about the behaviors of an alpha, and I thought, *Oh, my God! I should have seen this coming.*

I started to think about our trips to the dog park when we'd taken all three dogs. Noah would stand next to me; he didn't really seem to understand the concept of a dog park. Gabe would chase the ball. And Josee would play with all the other dogs. But Josee didn't know when to stop playing. Another dog owner would call, "Come on, Buster, we're going home."

Josee would be there pleading, "Please, please, please stay. Stay and play with me." The lady would be putting the leash on Buster, and Josee still didn't know to stop playing. She had lived in a crate all her life, so she was incredibly unsocialized, and her behavior was always over-the-top. No wonder she didn't have any limits.

I told the behaviorist, "She would never stop. She had no boundaries."

Josee had been in training to become a therapy dog, but she never got through that, or through obedience training. She was fine with people, but over time would try to dominate the pack. I said, "I would never want her to hurt a person." But the behaviorist thought she was just an alpha dog that would do better in a home without any other animals. The rescue center posted Josee's info online, and within two days, a lady from Deer Valley, Arizona, adopted her. It was right around Thanksgiving, so that worked out well for Josee.

I carried a great deal of guilt for a long time that I had brought a dog into our home that had tried to harm Gabriel. That incident made him extremely fearful of any dog running up to him. He seemed to experience the dog version of post traumatic stress disorder for quite some time. Though he was never aggressive, if a dog came running toward him, he would back up and bark at it, as if to say, "You're in my space." He never really got over that completely. Dogs learn by experience, the good ones as well as the bad ones.

I said, "Never again. Never again am I going to bring a dog into our family." I was that traumatized.

* * *

In 2007 I got "the call" from my friend Rebecca, who headed up our local Weimaraner Rescue. I knew her pretty well and loved her dearly for all she's done for the breed. She'd never heard about my Josee incident, so she said innocently, "I want to talk to you about this dog I have."

"No!"

"But you have to at least give…"

"No! Rebecca, I'm not doing that again."

She kept at it. "Can I say one thing?"

"What?!"

"I have a big one here, a big Weim named Jack, and I want to tell you that I see one like this every ten years. He is a kind soul with a sad story. He would make a great therapy dog."

Oh, no. Here we go again. I said, "Okay, tell me more."

She continued, "He was turned in to the ASPCA in Albany, New York, because he blew out both of his knees. Evidently, Jack's family couldn't afford the surgery." Ruptured ACL ligaments are not particularly common in Weimaraners, but now that I know Jack, I can see that happening. He'll go and go and go, flying around the yard. I now know from experience that he'd probably hurt his knees doing something crazy.

"I want you to come and meet him," Rebecca pleaded. I later learned that while Jack was at the ASPCA in Albany, they repaired one of his knees. Then a local man saw Jack and wanted to adopt him. The man was moving to Arizona, though, and wanted to take Jack with him. He signed the paperwork promising that he would have Jack's other knee repaired after he got situated in Arizona. A month later, Jack showed up at a Phoenix veterinary clinic to be euthanized, because this man's new wife wouldn't let him spend the money to repair Jack's knee.

The vet said, "I am not going to euthanize this beautiful and otherwise healthy dog." Someone from his clinic's staff called Weimaraner Rescue, and Rebecca picked him up. Jack lived there with her and fourteen other Weimaraner rescues. It was December 2006, and the volunteers decided to wrap gifts at Border's Bookstore to raise funds for Jack's surgery. They took in $3,000, and Jack had surgery on his other knee. When Rebecca initially called me, Jack was rehabbing from this surgery.

I agreed to "look" at Jack and went out to see him. Solo. I told Mike this time, since last time with Josee, things hadn't turned out so well. I met Rebecca and Jack at a park. There was petite little Rebecca with the biggest, lankiest, most beautiful Weimaraner I'd ever seen. He was tall and stately, with these amazing long ears, just beautiful.

I've read that Weimaraners from Europe tend to be taller and leaner than they are here in the States. As you move west, the breed tends to get smaller. They thought this might be the case with Jack, in that he was from New York. To this day, when we're at the park, people continually keep coming over to pet him. He was a bit underweight when we met him, but for rehab purposes, that was great. What those volunteers did for Jack saved his life.

I was, of course, in love again. I heard no internal voice saying, "What are you doing? Remember what happened last time?" I just knew this gentle giant was for us. I went home and said to Mike, "He's the most handsome Weim I have ever seen. And his temperament is beautiful."

The next day, we took Gabriel and Noah to meet Jack at the park. We all went for a walk, and they got to know each other. Everything went well; they were on neutral territory meeting a laidback new friend. We drove home, a fifty-mile trek, one way. Mike was smitten as well, so we decided to give it another try. Jack needed a home, and his story was so heartwarming that it really was an easy decision. I got back in the car after dropping off Mike and the dogs at home. Jack had been crate trained, so I wanted him to have a comfortable place to stay. On my way to the pet store, I counted on my fingers how many homes poor Jack had had in his short life. Mike, Gabriel, Noah, and I would make his fifth home, his forever home. I bought the crate and went to pick up our new boy.

* * *

I wondered, *What's different about this time from the time with Josee?* Nothing specific; I think it was just my intuitive sense that this would be different. Looking back on Josee, there had been subtle signs that she had no boundaries. One time when I was playing with her, she picked up a plastic water bottle and began running around the house, looking for some fun. So I played around, trying to get the bottle from her. Gabe saw us having a good time and decided he wanted to join in. All of a sudden, Josee got mad at Gabe for wanting to play, too. Mike said to me,

"That's your fault. You got everyone all hyped up."

I thought Mike might be right, but nothing more happened, so we dismissed it. *Mike's right — I got everyone all hyped up.* Looking back, though, the dog park incident with Buster had also been a red flag.

I had no proof, but I felt things were different with Jack. I hadn't gone to a rescue to get Josee; she'd had a home. Jack had nobody. He was living in a rescue that does a great job, but he didn't have a family. It was exciting to realize I had rescued my first dog! The difference for me was that I felt I had to take Gabe when I did because someone else might have come along that afternoon and bought him. When you're buying a purebred dog, things become a little competitive. I felt the same way with Noah. He was the last puppy of the litter, and someone was scheduled to look at him that afternoon.

Adopting Jack from a rescue was something of a shift for me, personally, because I saved an animal that no one else wanted. I saved a life, versus being part of a competition to buy a puppy. Rescuing him changed me forever. I think Jack was meant to be in my life to teach me the merits of giving a home to a living being that otherwise wouldn't have had one.

When you think about it, Gabe and Noah grew up pretty privileged, noses in the air: "I'm here, and everything is mine."

Jack, on the other hand, marvels at each new day. Every day, he greets life with the attitude of, "Hooray, hooray — another day!" Whether that appreciation is something I intuitively see in him, or he really is that way, he's definitely different from the other dogs.

After leaving Rebecca's, I arrived home with Jack. We decided to let the dogs meet as we walked them down the street. Mike brought Gabriel and Noah out the front door on leashes. Immediately, they barked at Jack, and he was visibly intimidated by them. Still, all five of us went walking down the street together. Eventually all three dogs were walking in an orderly fashion, so we decided to put them in our backyard, leashes off. I noticed a lot of positioning right away, but Jack isn't an alpha. He's not really a leader — he's just happy to be alive.

As Jack settled in over the next couple days, I noticed that he and Noah treated Gabriel as the patriarch of the family. Jack and Noah would allow him to go outside first. They always yielded to Gabe — not because he demanded it, but out of respect.

GABRIEL'S ANGELS

* * *

Noah is ten-and-a-half years old now. We know that someday, we will have to get Jack another dog. He loves little dogs. It's as if Jack believes that all little dogs are puppies, and he has to care for them because they are so small. Conversely, all big dogs — whether it's a puppy or an adult dog — frighten big Jack.

I said to Mike the other day, "Someday, Jack will have a little dog. It will be a rescue, but Jack needs to have a little dog. And it will be our first little dog." We're just sure it would be good for Jack. We know of Marley, a Weimaraner, who has a teeny little Chihuahua pal named Lulu with markings like a Holstein cow. They are so cute together.

* * *

One day, not long after adopting Jack, I heard a popping sound in one of his knees, so I took him to see a veterinary surgeon. Jack had had the ligaments in his knees replaced, but not a full-blown knee replacement. This is understandable, since both his surgeries were performed while he was a rescue dog without a family. It was recommended that we pursue a TTA for Jack's knee. This is a surgical repair done by putting a plate in the knee. It greatly slows the progression of arthritis that tends to occur when the knee ligaments are repaired. Jack was already showing some signs of advanced arthritis, and he was still a young dog. In October 2006, we decided to have the TTA done.

Jack stayed at the veterinary hospital for a few days, and when I went to pick him up he had a huge cast on his leg. Jack needed 24/7 monitoring — and you should have seen me trying to lift him. He's probably about a hundred pounds. Lifting him in and out of the car was a real back breaker. If I didn't do it correctly, he and I would go spinning around — me trying to hold onto him, and him spinning on his one good leg. So it was interesting, to say the least. But Mike helped when possible, and we were very careful with him.

Jack was healing slowly and steadily after the surgery, be he never really seemed to recover completely. One Sunday night in November, I noticed him lying in his dog bed shaking. I asked Mike, "What's wrong with Jack?" He told me the shaking had just started.

I sat up with Jack all night and drove to the clinic at seven o'clock the next morning, gently guiding him inside. He walked into the clinic and collapsed in the reception area. I screamed, "Something's wrong with Jack! Something's wrong!"

Immediately the receptionist yelled, "Jack Gaber collapsed! Jack Gaber collapsed!" After Jack was admitted, he was at first confined to the isolation ward because they thought he might have canine influenza or pneumonia — some kind of upper-respiratory illness. His eyes were goopy, and he wasn't breathing well. They did tests and ruled out a canine upper-respiratory problem. They did every test possible, and he came back positive for Valley Fever. Lucky Jack. He'd been in Arizona six months, and already he'd contracted Valley Fever. He probably stepped off the plane from New York and caught it with one sniff.

We wondered if the problem might be a Valley Fever lesion, because his leg still wasn't healing properly. That culture came back negative, so it wasn't a Valley Fever lesion. The testing finally revealed that Jack had a latent staph infection in his knee. He had MRSA (methicillan resistant staph aureus), a "super bug" that kills some humans who contract it. It is resistant to antibiotics, except one that is very expensive. We agreed to use that drug to save Jack, but it wasn't as simple as that. At one point, his white cell count was 75,000. Normal is around 10,000. He was put on a slow intravenous drip of the antibiotic for five to six hours every day.

Jack spent about a month in Intensive Care. Throughout this ordeal, Mike and I decided that if Jack wanted to live, we wanted him to live, so we were in it to the end. That's why one of Jack's nicknames is "Kitchen Remodel!" I have my beloved Jack, along with my same old kitchen.

During his stint in Intensive Care, I received a call that Jack had blown a pulmonary embolism. They told me he was in the oxygen chamber, and I should come right down. After it looked as if Jack would pull through, I dubbed his stay in the oxygen chamber as "Jack in the Box." Each time he went in for a treatment, that was what the technicians called it. I visited every day, from three in the afternoon to seven at night. I sat with him and force fed him, repeatedly asking the vet, "Are we doing anything more than just keeping him alive?"

"Pam," the vet said, "I can tell you that he's fighting. He's fighting every step of the way. I would tell you if I thought we were just prolonging his life artificially. Now, of course the cost is there, and if the cost is why you don't want to do it..."

That's what is known as economic euthanasia. I understand that many people do not have the means to take on such a financial responsibility. Fortunately for Jack, we had the means to do it. I acknowledge that even if some people had the means, they might not spend that much on the care of their animal. But that just isn't me. How could I be willing to keep him alive for $10,000, but put him to sleep when the cost reached $15,000? During Jack's hospitalization, Mike and I put the cost out of our minds and focused on getting him better. You do what you've got to do. And we still have Jack, so that's good.

* * *

I suspect that in Jack's previous life as a rescue dog, he was never quite sure when his next meal was coming. To this day, he always eats quickly and looks around for more. Watching him reminded me of some of the children at Crisis Nursery. Those living in violent homes might not be fed very regularly, so they would eat a lot at the nursery and hide food, just in case it might be a while until their next meal. I remember noticing little Danny's pockets bulging with cookies. When I asked him why, he said, "Because Miss Pam, maybe later there won't be any more food, and I will be hungry. I will share my cookies with you, though." Their reality could be just heartbreaking.

This is why, when Jack began to refuse food while he was in Intensive Care, we were very concerned. Trying to get him to eat was quite a challenge. The only thing he would eat was Gerber baby food hotdogs. The vet bought cases of the things at Costco, and I fed them to him every night. When he refused those, I diluted high-calorie canned dog food and force-fed him with a large syringe. Finally his metabolism evened out, and he began to eat on his own. Today Jack is a registered therapy dog. He inspires the teenagers he visits to believe that they, too, will one day overcome the odds and find their forever home.

At one point, while the eight-hour antibiotic drip was being administered, Jack decided to lie upside down. This caused the antibiotic to travel outside the vein and into the tissue, causing tissue necrosis. He now sports a big pink scar on his right front leg. The scar is a badge of honor for him and a reminder of his bravery. And it's always a conversation starter with the new teens he visits.

* * *

Finally Jack was ready to come home! All his tests were normal. It would be a test of Mike's fortitude to write that check to bust Jack out of the hospital. My favorite receptionist asked, "Is your husband going to knock himself out on our marble counter when he sees the final bill?"

I said, "I don't know — maybe. But we're in a hospital, so if it has to happen, this is a good place."

When we checked Jack out of the hospital, he was a mere seventy-two pounds; he had lost about a quarter of his weight. I was confident we could get the weight back on him, though, because his appetite was back to normal. The hospital had a bon voyage party for him. Jack walked down the hallway with all the employees and veterinarians clapping and cheering for him. He ate it up and proudly made his way into my arms. "Let's go home, Jack," I said.

He really is something special, and he really has a beautiful story about a dog who found his forever home. He inspires hope in the kids that the same is possible for them.

CHAPTER TEN

Why Pet Therapy Works

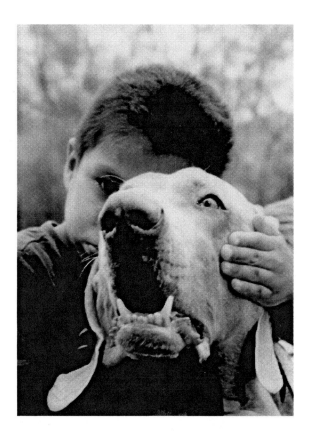

The term "link," as coined by the American Humane Society, defines a substantiated correlation between child abuse, animal cruelty, and other crimes against humans. It is undeniable that animal abuse is often one of the early signs of families in crisis, and it's highly predictive in identifying children at risk for abuse and becoming potential abusers. This type of violence is insidious, cyclical, and is passed on from one generation to the next, without some form of intervention.

Current research shows that children who are abused are more likely to become abusive adults. However, the strongest predictors of subsequent violence and abuse can be changed.

Gabriel's Angels' pet therapy program addresses the root cause of the social problem by treating the symptoms and cause of the problem and intervening in this perpetuating cycle. We work on improving healthy core behaviors that are critical to normal childhood development, focusing on improving empathy, self-esteem, trust, compassion, respect, and encouraging nurturing behavior in a safe environment. These behaviors are also proven to interrupt the cycle of violence.

— **Gabriel's Angels 2010 Annual Report**

Once I learned that children need seven core behaviors to be successful in life, I began to notice how naturally the children demonstrated them when they were with a therapy dog. Abused, abandoned, and neglected children need to master these core behaviors in order to exit the cycle of violence, so why couldn't we deliberately teach the behaviors through interactions with a therapy dog?

Violent behaviors are cyclical. Frequently, the adults in the lives of these children are either unable to express or don't know how to teach their children empathy. They don't teach them to nurture, probably because they never learned it themselves. Likewise with trust, compassion, self-esteem, respect, and affiliation. No one taught Mom or Dad those things, and they can't teach their children what they don't know, so the cycle continues. The social change we're trying to implement is growing the first generation of non-abusing, nonviolent people.

I asked myself, "How can we instill these core behaviors in these kids by bringing the child into closer contact with an animal?" Were we creating the kinds of lasting changes that could actually intervene in the cycle of violence? I thought so, but one would expect me to think that, as the founder of the organization. In 2003, we applied to St. Luke's Behavioral Health for a $6,000 grant for our very first formal program evaluation. This would be a concrete way of determining whether our program was as effective as we perceived it to be. We received the funding — and then I started to worry. *Suppose our program does nothing for these kids?*

The Tucson, Arizona, firm we hired performs formal program evaluations for human services agencies. They developed a five-point Likert scale that the staffs at our client agencies could use to rate the development of core behaviors they saw in their children. The results told us that we were making an impact, even though pretty much all we were doing was having a therapy team — one dog and one human — show up. Yet our facilities told us they saw an increase in these core behaviors that are known to intervene in the cycle of violence.

I was very happy to know we were making an impact, but at this stage, we were more or less doing it on accident. I wanted to know how we could do it on purpose. My goal was to create a program through which we could intentionally teach the core behaviors.

I convened several child welfare experts in our boardroom and asked, "What else can we do? Here's what we're doing now. What else can we do?" The ideas that came from these people were amazing. They discussed how children who regularly witness violence or who have been abused and neglected are frequently desensitized to violent acts. Sometimes, they begin abusing animals because they have no reverence for life. So maybe it would be a good idea to have them use a stethoscope to listen to the heartbeat of the therapy dog. When a five-year-old, a ten-year-old, even a fifteen-year-old hears the heartbeat of that animal, it builds empathy and helps them understand that the dog is a living being that they should love back. We now include a stethoscope in all of our activity kits.

One time, four-year-old Axel said, "Hey, Gabriel's heartbeat sounds like bubbles!" Cute. After listening to the dog's heartbeat, the kids listen to their own heartbeats. The goal is for them to draw a conclusion like, "Maybe Gabriel's not so different from me." Other goals are for them to develop a loving bond with animals and a reverence for all life.

The group of experts advised that seeing photos of the dog in his home environment would help the children deepen their relationship with the dog. Because children learn through pictures and stories, a photo album would give them the sense that, "Oh, an animal is a member of the family. He's like my brother, or my sister. I love him," which helps build empathy and compassion.

So we added a blank photo album to the kits to allow our teams to show their kids pictures of their animal living at home. Photos such as the dog getting a bath, going to the vet, or sleeping in his bed were recommended. I showed my kids at Crisis Nursery a photo of Gabriel sleeping on my bed, and they got such a kick out of that.

"Where's Gabriel?" I would ask.

"He's on your bed!"

Another important item in the kits is a Polaroid camera. A couple of important things happen with the camera. First, we take a picture of the child with the dog and give that picture to the child as a memento. Now they have a possession that belongs to them alone, something many of them have never had. Frequently, you'll see the photos thumbtacked above the kids' beds in the shelter.

The photo is also an opportunity to say, "Look, Joey. You're walking Gabriel. What a good job you did!" So the child now has a picture himself doing something well. Unfortunately, in their dysfunctional homes, all they tend to hear is, "You're just like your mother. You're just like your father. You don't do this right. You don't do that right." This photo offers the child proof that he can do something right. These pictures become a source of pride for the kids.

Each Gabriel's Angels therapy dog has its own trading card. They are like a baseball cards, with the dog's stats on the back, such as Favorite Treat, Favorite Trick, Shakes Right or Left, and a Humane Education quote on the back. Gabriel's card said, "I am a member of the family and want to be treated with kindness and respect." We give them to the kids so that they now have another possession and a memento of the visit. Sometimes these children are taken from their homes in the middle of the night in their pajamas. They have to share clothes and shoes and blankets, so they have nothing familiar, nothing that belongs to them alone. The trading card is a possession and a reminder of the unconditional love they experienced during their visit with the therapy team.

All of these activities take place through a program we call ACT: the Animals and Children Together Learning Project. We have three different kits, each one geared to a specific age level and with age-appropriate activities.

Noah's Tails is for children from infants to age five; *Penny's Pals* is for kids from six to twelve years; and *Gabe's Gang* offers a positive spin on "gang" for teenagers. The items in the kits vary according to the population we are visiting. Brushes are great for long-haired dogs, and all ages can brush the dog. When you're working with little children, sometimes the simplest things can mean the most. Now, a Weimaraner's fur is about an eighth-of-an-inch long, so it doesn't really need to be brushed. But the act of gently brushing Gabe helped the kids developed empathy, as well as teaching them to share and take turns.

However, I don't have a brush in the kit for Jack, my other Weimaraner who is still working as a therapy dog, because teenage boys can see there's no real benefit to brushing a dog with a short coat. For older kids' kits, we utilize bandage materials. It is amazing to see these hardcore boys work to gently bandage Jack's leg. Then, when he stands up, the bandage often falls right off because they used too light a touch. Of course Jack's not really hurt; we use it as an opportunity to teach the boys to gently compress when bandaging a dog — or anyone.

I contributed the activity of brushing the dogs' teeth. In each kit, we include a doggie toothbrush and toothpaste. The children get such a kick out of brushing the dogs' teeth, and no matter what age the child is, it builds empathy. Remember little Gabby, who was so sad to learn of Gabriel's passing? Her mom, Lissa, told me that Gabby enthusiastically began brushing her teeth more often because "that's what Gabriel does." I thought, *That is so cool.* Here we were, focused on building empathy, but the hygienic piece was a nice bonus outcome.

Nutrition is something else the dogs can teach the children. Gabriel always brought green beans and carrots with him in case he got hungry, and the children had the opportunity to feed him the snacks. Children love giving the dogs treats. It doesn't matter how old they are — from five to fifteen — when a child says, "Gabriel, sit," and he sits, you can see the child's self esteem rise. We started out bringing dog treats with us, but sure enough, Gabriel gained five pounds during his first year of visiting. It just makes sense, since he would sit, lie down, and shake fifty or sixty times each visit. So we switched over to veggies instead. Fortunately, he really did like them.

One little boy told me proudly, "Miss Pam, I eat my carrots just like Gabriel does!"

Another parent said to Gabriel one day, "So you're the dog that got Joey to eat his green beans!"

* * *

The activities in the kits help the children to learn self-regulation, which is vital, because kids who were not taught to self-regulate do not affiliate well. They might grab each other's brush, which gave me the opportunity to say something like, "Oh, Gabriel likes it when we share." Soon, they would all learn — and be willing — to stand patiently in line, waiting to share, because Gabriel asked them to do it.

Learning self-regulation (i.e., how to control one's emotions and behavior in certain circumstances) is really about self-awareness. When a two-year-old has a temper tantrum at the grocery store, they lack self-awareness, so they don't really care that everyone is staring at them. By age ten, however, a temper tantrum to get your way is inappropriate, but a child can only know that if they have learned to regulate their behavior because someone taught them to become self-aware.

Rather than utilize the animals as a reward, we've found that the therapy dogs usually bring out the best in the children. If we restrict a child who is having a hard day from visiting with the therapy dog, we lose the opportunity for the therapy dog to intervene in that child's bad day. There were occasional times when I had to say, "I'm sorry, but you have to walk away now," or "I'm sorry, but Gabriel's walking away now because you can't brush gently." It's an art, not a science. My number one priority was to keep Gabriel safe, and in ten years of visiting with these children, I never had an instance where he was in an unsafe situation.

* * *

Gabriel and I would frequently visit the children in an outside play area. This was the perfect opportunity to teach them to notice him panting and ask them, "So what does that mean?"

"He's hot!"

The simple act of noticing that Gabe was hot, and then caring enough to bring him water, was laying the groundwork for developing empathy, because it meant the child saw a need in another living being and cared enough to meet the need. "You have a need, and I care enough to help you." Filling a water bowl for Gabriel or admonishing another child, "Don't tug on Gabriel's leash," means the children are being mindful of someone's needs besides their own.

Gabriel wasn't the thirstiest dog in the world, so sometimes I had to cheat a little. If it was a chilly day, I would spike his water with a little chicken broth. He would have refused regular water but would happily drink the chicken-flavored stuff! I hated the thought of seeing the children's sad little faces when he would not drink the water, so it didn't bother me to nudge Gabe with a little extra motivation. And when they met his need (even if it was a bit manufactured), he would accept their gift, which resulted in a boost to their self-esteem — another important core behavior.

Building empathy is a big part of what we do. We can even teach teenagers to develop empathy. Murderers on death row who committed heinous crimes are nearly always sociopaths who lack empathy. I talk a lot about empathy because it's such an important building block for breaking the cycle of violence.

When working with the teens, I ask them, "So what do you need to do to have a dog? Can Gabriel go into the closet and get his food and put it in the bowl?"

"No!"

"OK, so you have to feed him. What else do you need to do to have a dog? Can Gabriel go turn on the water and get himself a drink?"

"No!"

"OK, so we have to give him water." We keep going until we create a list of nineteen or twenty things a good pet owner does. It becomes a contest, and in the end, it really instills in them an awareness of all the things involved in keeping and caring for an animal. (*See list on page 167.*)

* * *

Through the years, we've developed many activities, most of which depend on the age of the children. When walking a dog, the kids learn to share and take turns. When Gabe and I worked at the Crisis Nursery, I would say, "Gabriel really likes it when you share. Can you share and make him happy?" And these kids, who might otherwise have pushed and fought with each other to be first in line, would share.

The staff later told me, "They share because of Gabriel. They care enough about him to share." They might have gone into the classroom later and not shared so well, so the teachers would say, "Remember when you shared for Gabriel? Would you please do that now?" They would do things for Gabriel that they wouldn't do for each other. And even when he was not present, the staff used him as a reminder.

These anecdotes were good feedback, but we began to realize that we needed a more concrete measuring stick to be sure that the programs we implemented were working. In 2003, we began to perform a rigorous annual Program Evaluation that is based on objective and anecdotal input from the staff at the agencies we serve. The people who work with the kids every day are the ones who tell us, "Over time, Tommy has developed more compassion. Over time, Susie finally learned to trust." It's like that story about Tatiana. Every person and everything she'd ever trusted had led to disappointment, so she wasn't going to trust Gabe, either. Gabe was her first relationship with someone who came through for her on a consistent basis.

We perform the Program Evaluation for two reasons. The main reason is that it makes us a better organization. It helps us determine the areas where we can improve. The second reason is that funders want to see programmatic outcomes from the organizations they invest in. We evaluate our short-term, midterm, and long-term outcomes. Our short-term outcomes are determined by the impact the therapy dog had on a child while the visit occurred. Did the child experience an hour-and-a-half of outward focus? Did that child have such a great time that he momentarily forgot about his circumstances and got lost in the moment? That's a beautiful short-term outcome. It's not about social change; it's just a nice short-term outcome.

The mid-term outcome is the development of the core behaviors known to intervene in the cycle of violence. Then our long-term outcome is that all the children develop a reverence for life. That is the long-term vision, that they have and display a reverence for life. All the work leads to the long-term outcome, but we excel in the short-term and mid-term outcomes because we've taken the time to evaluate our progress.

Along the way, we have learned what works and what doesn't work. Here is a personal example. One day, I thought it would be interesting to put five leashes on Gabriel's collar so that several children could walk him at the same time. I had one of the leashes; four of the kids had the others. But having that many children trying to navigate with Gabriel was a disaster. One child tripped while the other kids kept walking. Everyone was pulling Gabriel in a different direction, and he looked at me like, "What did I do to deserve *this*???!"

Another thing we've learned over time is that our adult volunteers do not think like children. We may go in thinking, "OK. They brought Gabriel water last week," or "They brushed Gabriel's fur last time I was here. They must be tired of that. What else can we do?" The biggest mistake a therapy team can make is to assume that the children are bored with an activity. Children delight in learning what to do and then doing it well. In fact, it's the repetition that builds the core behaviors in the children.

It may be similar, I think, to teaching a child you're parenting. A friend told me about having to teach her daughter the same lesson again and again. "So when the clerk hands you your change, you move out of the way to put it in your pocket or your little purse before you go out the door. Don't stand right there in front of the clerk. Move out of the way. Move out of the way. Move out of the way." My friend told me she must have said this a thousand times. And the first time her daughter moved out of the way, her response was, "Yeah!! She got it!" Building core behaviors in abused children is very similar. It's all about the lessons and the opportunity to practice again and again.

Not to mention that there are one hundred sixty-eight hours in a week. Think back to being five years old, how slowly time passed. A week — that's how long it's been since they've brushed the dog or brought him water. The therapy team may spend two hours with the children, but in the week between visits, lots has happened. We constantly remind our volunteers, "You're not a kid, and they're not bored." We adults must remember that not only are they not getting tired of giving the dog water, they're also learning to remember to do it.

* * *

It's amazing and delightful to see the results our pet therapy teams are achieving, but we'll never really know the full extent of the impact we are having on these kids' lives — and the ripple effect the change in them is having on the community.

One day as we walked out to the nursery playground, the children were all gathered around a female staff member. As soon as they saw us, the kids left the woman and ran over to see Gabriel. The lady was squinting, as it was a sunny day, but beyond that, I sensed she was unhappy and attributed it to the fact that the kids had abandoned her to greet Gabe. She continued to sit there, scowling. I thought to myself, *Great. We certainly did not make a friend today. Gabriel, you are just too popular.*

We continued our visit, and it came time to leave. As we headed back into the building, the scowling lady was waiting for us. Her face had softened somewhat, so I thought maybe it had just been the bright sun getting in her eyes. As I walked up to her, she said, "I want to tell you something."

Ooooo-kay... I thought. *What could this be about?*

She said, "You really have no idea the impact you're making on these kids. Can I tell you about the morning we had today? It was crazy and chaotic, and the children were so hyper. The minute Gabriel got here, everything changed. They are now calm and happy. I want to thank you and Gabriel for coming today." When I'd seen her scowling, she'd probably just been exhausted, but I had interpreted it differently. I told her how much I appreciated her feedback; it really cemented for me how Gabriel's gentle presence could turn the nursery into an oasis of serenity, not only for the kids, but for the staff, too.

I wish the staff would regularly give us feedback, both positive and negative, but they are busy and don't always have time. Unless something exceptionally noteworthy occurs or a volunteer shares it with us, we don't hear too much about the day-to-day visits. That's what makes our formal Program Evaluations so powerful: we specifically ask the agencies' staffs to provide us with anecdotes and observations so that we can better understand our impact. It's how I learn about the child who spent all morning in timeout, crying and miserable, but the minute the pet therapy team got there, that kid had a great rest of the day.

* * *

Animals are part of many children's lives from the time they are born. From Barney to Blues Clues to the family dog, animals romp through our children's experiences. Doing this work, I learned that more than one-half of all American children live with pets, and they are more likely to grow up with a pet than with both parents. A Google search for "children and animal books" returned more than 29,000 results. Many children report confiding in their pets, and a study of seven- to ten-year-olds found that children with pets in the household were as likely to talk to their pets about feeling sad, angry, lonely, or happy as with their siblings. According to another study, interviews with Michigan children between the ages of ten and fourteen revealed that seventy-five percent of them turned to their pets when they were upset. The unconditional attentiveness of a dog can offer limitless understanding to a child. In my youth, my dog's accepting and uncritical demeanor made me feel comfortable in sharing my feelings with him. For older children, unlike a blankie or stuffed animal, it is never suggested that they outgrow their pets in the name of maturity.

I believe that the loss of a pet, for some of these kids, is their first experience in life of a healthy loss. Of course, this depends on how the parents handle it. I've learned that adults should never say, "We had to put Spot to sleep," because you could be creating a child who will never want to go to sleep again. The way adults handle loss with kids is important — the best thing is to be honest about the loss, guiding them as much as possible through the process of grieving and experiencing the pain.

When I was five years old, my parents told me that my St. Bernard had not adjusted well to my new little brother, and they'd sent him to live on a farm. That's what they told me, and I had no reason not to believe them. It may sound impossible, but I believed until I was twenty-one that my beloved Stashu had gone to live on a farm.

I was teaching some veterinary technicians a class in medical terminology, and somehow that topic came up. Perhaps we were talking about euthanasia. I told the students what I'd always believed, that when I was young, my dog had gone to a farm because he had not adjusted well to the arrival of my baby brother. A smart, bold student raised her hand and said, "He didn't go to a farm."

"Excuse me, what are you talking about?" I asked.

She said very matter-of-factly, "Your dad told you he took your dog to a farm?"

"Yeah…"

"He didn't take your dog to a farm — he put your dog to sleep!"

You might think I'd have been embarrassed, but my only thought was, *Oh, my God!* When I got home that night, I called my dad and said, "Tell me about Stashu. Remember when I was little, and you told me you took him to a farm because he didn't like Stevie?" My dad was quiet, and then I knew the truth — he hadn't taken Stashu to a farm. He did what he thought was best, but he never let me experience the loss. I was only five, but he deprived me of an important lesson that was delayed until much later in my life.

* * *

Over the years, we have had therapy dogs pass away or retire. When a dog retires, we have a retirement party so the children will have closure. The children make cards to honor their dog. I remember we held a party for another dog where Gabriel worked, and a cute little girl came up to me and asked, "Did you know, Miss Pam, that Mac re-tiwerd. He re-tiwerd." She was so cute, trying to say such a big word.

"Yes, I heard that Mac retired."

"Yes, he re-tiwerd."

We hold the retirement parties because we don't want Mac to just go away and never show up again. That would be as if he had dumped on these fragile kids.

Then we have situations when dogs pass away. When a therapy dog passes away, we ask the owner to visit the children for a closure event, so they can present the adult with handmade gifts or cards that they made. Initially the owner is usually hesitant, because they are still grieving the loss of their dog. I can speak to this one from personal experience. Often we hear, "Oh, I can't do it. I can't. It would just be too hard."

But we gently insist, "We need you to do it for the kids." We've found, since we've implemented these closure ceremonies, that they have become as healing for the volunteers as they are for the children.

CHAPTER ELEVEN

When God Winks

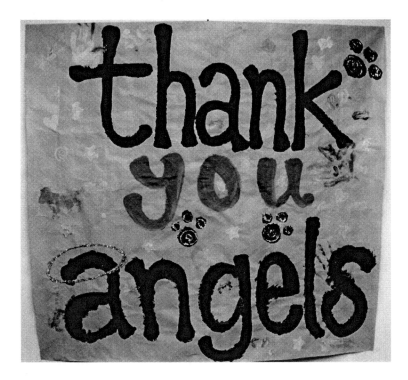

Early on, as I struggled to learn the art of raising money, a local organization chose Gabriel's Angels to be the recipient of the proceeds from
their Casino Night. It was a fancy shindig held at the Scottsdale Galleria,
an upscale indoor mall. I took Gabriel, and a few other therapy teams
were there. We encountered a challenge when we found that the only
way we could enter the venue was by going down an escalator. *Just
great*, I thought. I looked at Gabriel and said, "You can to do this." He

walked to the steps, surveyed the situation, and simply got on and rode the escalator down. At the bottom, he walked over to the "up" side and went right back up! So up we went, and down we went. He had a ball.

As Gabriel's Angels was in serious need of funding, this group seemed like a lifesaver. They indicated to us that the funding would be "substantial." *Finally*, I thought. It was a long night for the dogs, but well worth the effort to raise some much needed capital. I received a call two weeks later to tell me the organization would like to present a check to our agency. *How exciting! Our very first real check presentation!*

They invited Gabriel to the cocktail party so he could mingle with the crowd. Notice I didn't say that I was invited. It was almost as though he was the celebrity, but because he couldn't drive himself, I was always included as the "plus one." At the end of the conversation, they told me the amount of this substantial contribution: two hundred dollars. I was dumbfounded. I didn't mean to be ungrateful, but honestly, what could we do with two hundred dollars? That might get us a couple inkjet cartridges and a case of envelopes. I tried to not sound disappointed and thanked them for their efforts on our behalf.

The evening of the check presentation arrived, and I realized my SUV was in the shop. I had rented a sedan that happened to have leather seats, but didn't even think of it until it was time for us to leave for the event. I said to Mike, "This is not good," as Gabriel had never ridden in anything but an SUV. I arrived home late from the office and said to Gabriel, "Come on! We have to go, we have to go!" I was tired and a bit deflated about having to go out to yet another event to pick up this "substantial amount of money."

Gabriel stared at me, as if to say, "No, I am not going, because you haven't thrown the ball yet. It's five o'clock and you are supposed to throw the ball. Remember the ball, the one you taught me to fetch?" But somehow I convinced him that we could play later, and we headed out to the car. I opened up the door to the rental car, and he looked at me like, "What is this?"

"Get in the backseat!"

Gabe just looked at me: "I'm *not* getting in that backseat."

"Please, Gabriel. You have to. We need to do the right thing and pick up the check." So he got in. And there he was, standing on the leather, which I envisioned his claws completely destroying. Somehow, he managed to sit, though he looked quite uncomfortable. I took off, and when I looked back, he had ended up with his butt on the seat and his front paws on the floorboard. Gabe had settled in, but I was still feeling sorry for myself, wondering how I could grow this agency to meet the demand for our pet therapy services. Driving all over town for two hundred dollars wasn't going to cut it — that was for sure.

I thought to myself, *I don't know what I'm doing. This was built up to be a big event. How could I have so misread the possible outcome? If we don't start raising money, what's going to happen? Mike and I can't fund this forever, and it won't be a charity anymore. I don't know what I am doing. This is a bunch of baloney. I don't know how to raise money. And, look, we're at the Country Club!* I wasn't really ready to throw in the funding towel at this point; I don't think I ever would have. But I admit I was discouraged. However, I had to put on my game face now. The pity party was officially over.

Gabriel was wagging his tail in anticipation of getting out of the backseat. We walked into the country club, and the general manager came over to see Gabriel. They were old friends, having met at a prior event. Then upstairs we went to the big cocktail party. This was a business networking event, and Gabe was wearing his therapy vest and mingling with the crowd. He could work the crowd like nobody's business and made every person he greeted feel like a million bucks. I heard comments like, "Oh, Gabriel, you are a lucky dog to be here tonight!" And they were all giving me high-fives, which made me think, *I certainly must have misunderstood the amount of tonight's donation. That will teach you, Gaber.*

The announcement came from the stage, "May we please have Gabriel come to the stage?" *What am I, chopped liver?* I thought. Gabriel and I approached the stage, everyone in the crowd still high-fiving me. The president of the organization spoke into the mic, "We are so happy to be able to support your organization, Pam. The work you do it is fantastic. Will you please say a few words?"

I spoke about our agency and thanked everyone for their generosity. The president handed me an envelope, a sealed envelope. I said, "Thank you," and as we left the stage, the crowd high-fived me some more. We left soon after, and while we walked to the parking lot, I said, "Dang, Gabriel. I must have totally misunderstood the amount, as everyone was so excited to present me with all this money they raised." My bleak mood was gone and I felt very happy. I got in the car where it was dark and no one could see me tear open the envelope. I looked down: two hundred dollars. And I thought, *Just stop whining and be grateful.*

On the way home, I called Mike. "I don't know what I'm doing. I don't even know how to raise money. I am so tired. I can't be chasing two hundred dollars. I can't do it like that. I don't know what I'm doing."

Gabriel sat quietly in the back, probably thinking, "Hey, I did my part!"

When we got home, Mike was standing there in the kitchen, and he just handed me a glass of wine. He didn't say anything. Again I said, "I just don't know what I am doing."

"You know, it just takes time," he reassured me. "Don't worry — it will all work out." He is and always has been my biggest supporter. I, of course, was still feeling pretty bad about this two hundred dollar donation.

* * *

We had about twenty-five therapy teams at this time, so we were definitely on our way and knew we didn't want to call it quits. But the therapy teams have always been the easy part of this project. Great people and great dogs who want to help kids came out of the woodwork to find us. That resource engine, on the other hand, can kill you until you figure it out. We were growing but still small, and I was still working out of our house.

The day after the big check presentation, I received a phone call from a guy who said, "Hi, Pam. My name is Louie, and I'm calling from a health benefits consulting firm."

"Hi, Louie. How are you?"

"Doing well," he said. "I have an employee who was at last night's event at the Phoenix Country Club."

At this point, my eyes were rolling, and I was thinking, *Ohhhhh, great!* But I managed to get polite words to come out of my mouth. "Oh, really, Louie?"

Louie continued, "Yes, and she brought me the information packet about your organization that she received last night. The reason I'm call-

WHEN GOD WINKS

ing is that we hold a golf tournament every year."

By now I might have been sighing audibly. *Louie,* I remember thinking, *I'm not going down that road again.*

Louie, bless his heart, was still talking: "We've held these tournaments for organizations you provide pet therapy to: Crisis Nursery, Homeward Bound, Sojourner Center, Boys and Girls Clubs ... I see they're all on your list. That's pretty coincidental. Now, I can't make the decision today, but I would really like to submit Gabriel's Angels as the recipient for this year's tournament because I think it would be a slam dunk for our committee to choose you."

I said, "OK," still thinking, *Big deal. It's going to be another two hundred dollars.*

And then he got my attention. "This event will raise between $20,000 and $25,000 for your organization."

"Excuse me? Would you say that again, Louie?"

"Between $20,000 and $25,000 — maybe more."

I thanked him and quickly hung up the phone. "YAY! Wooooo-weeeee!" Gabriel had been sleeping in my office and opened one eye to make sure I was okay. I looked up at the sky and said, "You got me," because I suddenly realized how severely my wherewithal had been tested.

I call situations like these, "when God winks." I truly felt like God was winking at me, saying, "Don't give up. Everything is going to be okay." Of course, the money wasn't in hand yet, but I knew the organizations this group had supported in the past, so it sure seemed to have legitimacy.

They did indeed choose Gabriel's Angels as the beneficiary of their next golf tournament. We took about five therapy teams out to the course on the day of the event to sell raffle tickets and greet the golfers at the holes. Gabriel and I were assigned to staff one of the holes — in retrospect, not the best job for a ball-aholic. True to form, Gabe grabbed one guy's golf ball in his mouth as it rolled past him. "No!!" I yelled. "Drop it!!" And he did. The golfer didn't see it happen, and I never told.

A dinner concluded the day's events. They auctioned off breakfast with Gabriel as an additional fundraiser. The winner was a very nice lady who had breakfast at Starbucks with Gabe at a later date. It was really cute. And they raised $26,000 for us.

GABRIEL'S ANGELS

That day, I learned never to doubt the circle of philanthropy. It's tough, though, because once you're inside of it, you can't control it as much as you would like. In my previous career, we would package a product and launch it. Philanthropy doesn't work that way. You can't always see the threads and connections.

So would I give back that original "measly two hundred dollars?" Absolutely not, because that two hundred turned into $26,000. And that's why, when my staff is out speaking or attending events and they say, "It wasn't very good," I remind them of this story and they instantly get it. Arriving at the golf tournament by way of Casino Night needed to happen so I could understand the giving circle. You have to be pretty open and spiritually aligned to grasp that. I've read that many for-profit people never make it in the nonprofit sector because they're missing this element. Two huge keys to success are belief and openness, and they can't do it because they're used to always controlling the outcomes. They either adapt and learn, or they burn out.

CHAPTER TWELVE

Intervening in the Cycle of Violence

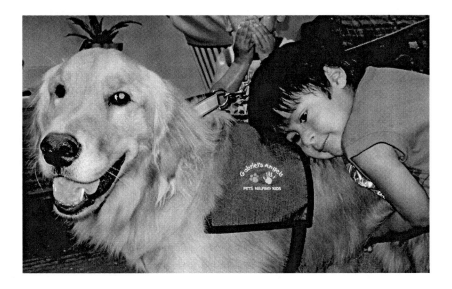

While there is definitely a correlation between children who suffer violence and abuse becoming abusers of both animals and people, I certainly don't want to imply that every child who has been abused or neglected is going to be an abuser, because that's simply not true. However, a strong relationship between the two behaviors does exist. And we've learned along the way that the core behaviors the Gabriel's Angels' therapy teams work to instill in our kids really do intervene to disrupt the cycle of violence.

GABRIEL'S ANGELS

Phil Arkow, animal-assisted therapy expert and the author of *Animal-Assisted Therapy and Activities: A Study, Resource Guide and Bibliography for the Use of Companion Animals in Selected Therapies*, has quite a bit to say on the subject:

> Experts in the arena of animal-assisted therapy began getting active around 1985 in an area called "the link." This is an age-old concept that goes back several hundred years: children exposed to animal cruelty become desensitized to violence and are more likely to harm other animals and then to begin hurting humans. We've learned to recognize that animal abuse is part of the continuum of family violence.
>
> The more we explore this link, the more convincing the evidence becomes. In study after study, a high incidence of animal abuse is found in the childhood histories of violent criminals, and embedded within the constellations of child abuse and domestic violence. Battered pets are a significant component of family violence and a strong indicator of other social problems and the propensity toward interpersonal violence. Generally speaking, when people are abused, animals are at risk, and when animals are abused, people are at risk.
>
> It has become apparent that the old model wasn't inclusive enough; we now recognize that it takes all of us to form a more humane society. Today we are training officials and agency people to collaborate to address the prevention, identification, intervention, and treatment of all forms of family violence. We want people to look beyond their immediate areas of expertise and take notice. If they see violence in one area, there's a very real possibility that it also is occurring in other areas. Animal care and control, child protection, and domestic violence agencies are working together to:
> - Cross-train their caseworkers to recognize and report multiple forms of family violence.
> - Increase animal abuse prosecution and penalties.
> - Provide foster services for animals in the care of human victims of violence.
> - Educate the community about all forms of family violence.

I am proud to know that Phil Arkow validates the Gabriel's Angels model of teaching core behaviors to disrupt the cycle of violence. He explains, "Animals have an innate ability to cut through the clutter and reach the heart. Because they have such a calming influence and offer a sense of relief from the chaos of our world, they can teach us to be calm in the face of whatever is going on in our lives. Gabriel's Angels has broken ground dramatically in specifically targeting abused kids and using pets therapeutically. The success of such innovative thinking shows up in their work as significantly as anywhere."

* * *

Another thing we have learned about intervening in the cycle is that we're saving animals' lives. Once you build compassion, empathy, and reverence for the life of a dog, it's only logical that these kids will become less likely to abuse animals. David was a teenager in the group home Noah and I used to visit. During one visit, he pulled me aside and said "I want to tell you something." I was a bit hesitant, because when a teenage boy says he wants to tell you something, you never know what it might be.

But he was insistent, "No. I *have* to tell you something."

"Okay, David. What is it?"

"I get it," he said.

I was a bit confused, so I asked him, "What do you mean, you get it?"

Very quickly and quietly, he said, "I've abused animals before. But I understand now. I get it now and I will never do it again. I love Noah so much. He is so sweet and loves me so much. I never thought of animals as having feelings, and I was so frustrated when I did it. Really, I would never, ever hurt an animal again."

I didn't freak out or get upset. I just looked at him and said, "David, that's why we're here. I am so happy to hear you would never hurt an animal again." The odds are that once kids have been abused or neglected or witnessed violence, by the time they become teenagers, some will have abused animals. So David's disclosure wasn't shocking to me. It might have been to a newer volunteer, but by then I was familiar with the pattern of these boys' lives. Still, the fact that he told me was huge.

I'll never know precisely why David decided to confide in me that day. Maybe he told me because he felt guilty. He felt bad that he had hurt animals in the past, when he had such love for my animal. Now David understood that Noah was a living being who would shower him with unconditional love. Noah didn't know that he had hurt animals before. That's the beauty about animals — they don't judge. *Wow,* I thought. *Way to go, Noah!* I think David felt so open, so vulnerable, and so unconditionally loved that he felt he wanted to let me know he'd made a personal shift.

CHAPTER THIRTEEN

Money Magazine — We're Famous!

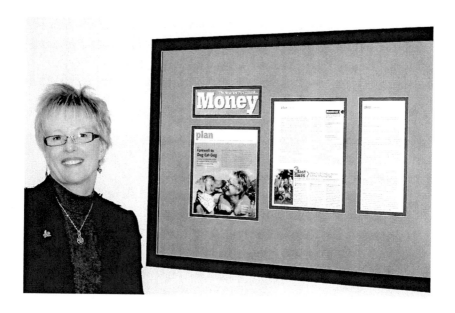

I remember the day Donna Rosato, a reporter from *Money* magazine, called me. One of my board members had heard that *Money* wanted to do a story about someone who had left the corporate world and found a life with meaning in the nonprofit sector. The reporter told me that the magazine receives a lot of editorial questions and comments like, "I'm working, but I don't know why I'm working," "I'm burned out," and "I want to leave and do something that matters with my life." Yet people felt they couldn't pursue these dreams because they were so comfortable in the lifestyles their current incomes were affording them.

We spoke a few times, but Donna never really made a commitment during those first few conversations. Finally she called me and said "I pitched my editor, and he wants to do it."

"Really!?" I was so excited.

Donna and I talked at length on the phone about the segment of the article that would be designed to educate people about planning for such a job shift. What could they do now that would enable them to join the nonprofit sector in five or ten years? Of course, I hadn't planned to create this agency while in Corporate America, but we did have the reserves that allowed me to start Gabriel's Angels. Some of the article focused on people who want to do this now, but it also touched on the fact that folks might be making plans to make this sort of change in the future. "I don't have the money now, so it's impossible," is a very real concern, which is why I recommend beginning to plan your exit strategy today.

As we were completing the interview portion, the magazine sent a photographer to Phoenix to get some pictures of our therapy teams, as well as Gabriel and me. It was a great experience, and I have fond memories of that photo session.

The first time I saw the article was in a bookstore. My sister comes to visit every year in July, and the article was due to be published in the August issue. We were in the bookstore when I mentioned, "I think that magazine should be out now. Let's look."

We found the August issue of *Money* magazine on the stand, and my sister started screaming across the store, "That's my sister! She's in this magazine!"

It wasn't a library, but most people were sitting or standing around quietly reading books, so they looked up at us like, "Why is that lady going crazy?"

"Mary," I hissed. "Stop it! Everyone is staring at us." She finally quit yelling and we bought at least six copies. At the checkout, she couldn't resist telling the cashier that I was in the magazine. My big sis sure was proud of me! That was on a Saturday. The following Monday, the phone calls and e-mails started flowing into the office. Lisa, our office manager, said, "There are a lot of e-mails."

"OK, I'll look at them," I responded.

She repeated, "There are a LOT of them."

She'd gotten my attention. "How many?"

"Like a couple hundred."

"You're kidding me!" She wasn't kidding.

Mary had flown home by then, and later that week she was checking her AOL e-mail account on her home computer. She looked up at her computer screen to see AOL's Top 5 Things for the day. The first was Brittany Spears. Eh. She looked down at the keyboard, then looked up at the screen again. There we were, Gabriel and I! Somehow, we'd made it to the front page of AOL. The phone calls and e-mails kept coming.

They were all questions like, "Ohhh, I just saw the article in *Money* magazine. How can we start a Gabriel's Angels in Virginia?" Or Denver? Or San Francisco? I even had an e-mail from Japan!

It was all very flattering, yet it taught me an important lesson. I will never shy away from national exposure, because I am not afraid of that, but when we hit the national media, we'd better be prepared for all the people and their dogs who will respond in such a positive manner. We returned every phone call and e-mail, because we really do have a dream of expanding nationally one day, and now we have the contacts when we are ready.

CHAPTER FOURTEEN

Right Human + Right Dog = Great Therapy Team

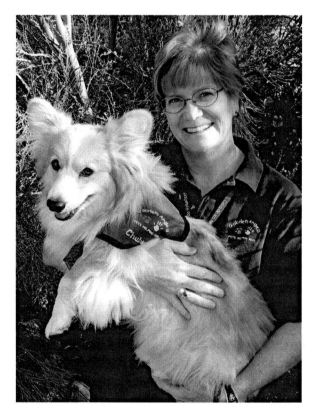

Matching the national trend, the average Gabriel's Angels volunteer is a woman between the ages of 30 and 55 who works outside the home and wants to make a difference in her community. One demographic we love and always want more of is male volunteers. These children have frequently witnessed violence committed by men, so they tend to stereotype all men as being violent. A man who is gentle and loving toward his pet is a great role model, because he teaches the children that not all men are harsh.

We've brainstormed about how to recruit more men into the program. We tend to find our volunteers where dogs and the people who love them congregate. In general, the primary caretaker of a pet in any family is the woman, so they may learn about us from a brochure in a veterinary hospital, a groomer, or pet store. Going forward, it would be great to have more men — and maybe do a targeted campaign: "Real men volunteer," or something like that.

People find out about Gabriel's Angels through word-of-mouth in the community, as well as through the media coverage we receive. If someone has a great dog or they want to be an assistant to a team, which we call a Helping Hand, they attend an info session at our office. We discuss how to know if you have the right dog for the job, how to become a registered therapy team, and everything else that's involved, e.g., fingerprinting and background check, reference check, specific training requirements, etc. That's about a two-month process, even if your dog is even slightly ready to get all the credentials needed. We also screen to make sure that all the dogs really like children. Therapy dogs work with all kinds of populations, so identifying the right group for the dog to work with is paramount, because not all dogs work well with children.

* * *

Gabriel's Angels works with therapy teams that are registered either through the Delta Society or Therapy Dogs Inc. The primary reason for this is insurance. Once a therapy team is registered with either of these organizations, they are covered under that organization's insurance policy. Interestingly, it's the insurance policy that gets therapy teams in the door in a lot of places, because the hospital, school, or social service agency can breathe a sigh of relief that the team is covered, in the event that anything should happen. At Gabriel's Angels, we prepare our teams so thoroughly that fortunately, up till now, we've never had to make any sort of an insurance claim.

Qualities we look for in our therapy dogs include, but are not limited to:
- Dogs that work well with children and are not timid.
- Dogs that are able to engage in the moment, and love to have little hands petting them.
- Dogs that are not *overly* friendly.

- Dogs that know how to greet their humans without jumping or barking.

The therapy dog evaluation process filters out most dogs that do not meet these qualifications; however, from time to time, a registered therapy dog is not accepted into our program because it gets overly excited around children or is too timid.

We also look for idiosyncrasies outside the spectrum, because sometimes a dog can test a lot better than their real-life experiences, or vice versa. Quite honestly, Gabriel did not test as well as he behaved in real life with the kids. It was as if he knew it was a test, and he was bored. At one evaluation, the tester asked me if Gabriel could show a little more enthusiasm. I upped my rhythm and became more animated, thinking it would no doubt rub off on him. He rolled his eyes as I said, "Come," got up from his Sit-Stay, and casually walked over to me. Actually, I wouldn't call it walking; it was more like he meandered over to me. In spite of this, we passed the evaluation and received our paperwork. It was then that he enthusiastically skipped out the door to the car.

* * *

Although we accept all sizes of dogs into our program, we're very careful with tiny dogs — for example a Chihuahua or Maltese — as we would not place a team like that with little children. Without meaning to, the children can be too rough. We have found that smaller dogs work well with pre-teen girls. Teen boys tend to like big dogs, so we usually place the larger breeds with that population. We also implemented a program called Gabe's Guests that brings in different therapy dogs to meet the children. A beefy teenage boy named Steven asked me if Gabriel's Angels had any poodles. I asked, "A standard poodle?"

"No," he said, "a teacup poodle." He went on to tell me that his Grandma had had a teacup poodle. When Steven had stayed at his Grandma's house because his parents were fighting, he would cuddle with the little dog. I suppose the lesson there is not to assume that all boys like big dogs.

Sometimes we have the right dog, but not the right person — these kids can spot a fraud a mile away. We are very careful which volunteers we place with teenagers. They must be genuinely interested in the children, without the tendency to be authoritative or dismissive.

From time to time, we encounter a volunteer who wants to visit the kids more than their dog does. They want so badly for their dog to work as a therapy dog, but sometimes we have to say to them, "Your dog is not enjoying this. He doesn't want to be here right now." In contrast, we had a lady a few years ago who had a darling dog, but she didn't want to have to sit on the ground at the children's level, because she didn't want to get dirty.

Hmm, I thought. *You want to work with kids, but you don't want to get dirty? I'm not so sure about that.* Even though someone could pass all the tests — obedience training, the therapy dog evaluation, and then the fingerprint and background check — they still might not be a good fit for our program.

It is so very important that we place a therapy team with the correct group of children. Some dogs work well with little children, some with pre-teens, and some with teenagers. Some humans would rather work with a particular age group. Gabriel loved the kids, and they loved him. He was the master at working with three- to five-year-olds. I discovered quite by accident, though, that he was not so good when visiting aging populations.

* * *

My mother-in-law, Rose, moved to an independent living facility near our home, and they have a floor that houses dementia residents. She's doing great on her own and lives independently, but she needed to be in a place where she could get additional care if she needed it. One of her favorite activities every day is going to the dining room to have her meals and socialize with the other residents. At lunch one day, she was talking to some of the staff about her "grand dog," Gabriel, and how he worked with children to help teach them compassion. "Gabriel this," and "Gabriel that." A staff member asked her if I would bring Gabe to see the Alzheimer residents. I had read about how well pet therapy works with older people and told the center staff I would be happy to take Gabriel for a visit.

Gabriel had never visited Alzheimer's patients before, but he worked so well with the children that I thought he would be just fine. When we first walked into the facility, he was okay, probably expecting that we were there to see some kids. As we rode the elevator to the fourth floor, I started to sense some hesitancy. A deep-seated communication tends to develop between the dog and its human when they work as a therapy team. My communication with Gabriel was unspoken, but it was as if I could read his mind. He greeted the residents, all the while looking up at me, as if to say, "What are we doing here?" I could that see he was unsure of exactly what to do, but I knew he would do what I asked of him.

I said in a calm, reassuring voice, "It's all right." We began to visit, and he loved the little lady in the wheelchair. She gently patted his head, and he was just fine with that. But within this unit were some patients who were a bit agitated, a few of whom were making some unusual sounds. One lady was carrying a baby doll, and Gabriel's eyes got big, thinking maybe she had brought it for him as a toy. At one point, he gently tried to remove the doll from her arms, and she became quite upset. He reluctantly released it, but clearly he was not in his element.

Everyone was thrilled to see him, but I could tell he was stressed out. They raved about Gabe and what an amazing dog he was. "Not his best work," I wanted to say, but we graciously thanked them for the invitation to visit and departed after he'd been petted by every resident. From that visit, I determined that the elderly were not his sweet spot.

I got him into the back of my car and told him, "I will never do that to you again. I promise." When they asked us if we'd come back, I declined, explaining that Gabriel's schedule with the children was too busy for him to fit in another visit. However, I did help them find a replacement dog that was much better suited to the elderly. The teaching point for me was that not every dog is great with every population.

Jan Hutchinson, the Delta evaluator, explains, "The dog and their handler have to figure out where they work best. But it's not just the dog — the team has to find out what works best for both of them." Some of our therapy dogs also wind up doing hospice work, visiting nursing homes, or working in hospitals. For others, like Gabriel, children are the population where they do their best work.

* * *

A lot of intensive work is done up front to ensure that we have a good placement. If we don't take that time, just randomly placing the teams anywhere, it might not be a good fit and the teams could decide to stop visiting. We avoid that at all costs, because we never want to give the children a reason or opportunity to say, "That dog disappointed me just like everybody else always has. I will never trust anyone again." That would compromise our ability to break through with them.

We have about a ninety-eight percent success rate in our placements, because we work really hard to find the right team for the job and then put them in the right venue with the right kids. We're working with fragile little lives that are just waiting for the next shoe to drop. As long as I have any input, it's not going to be our shoe.

We have learned that when teams work with older kids, the human becomes a more integral part of the process. When Gabe and I worked with the pre-school kids, I would ask them, "What's my dog's name?"

They'd scream, "Gabriel! Gabriel!"

Then I'd ask, "What's MY name?"

"We don't know!" they'd respond, or "Gabriel's mommy?"

When working with younger children, the dog is really so much more front and center. If a volunteer really thinks it's about them, that this experience is going to give them all the personal fulfillment *they* need, it's not as likely to happen with the littler people, because the little ones are all about the dog. As the kids get older, they notice there's a human there, too, and that a human is also kind of cool.

* * *

Once a therapy team has been accepted into our program, they have a one-on-one orientation with their volunteer coordinator. During this intensive training, the volunteer learns about post-traumatic stress disorder, attachment disorders, anger management issues — all the behaviors they are likely to see from these kids, and the reasons behind the behaviors. At times, our teams may encounter behaviors that can border on the unacceptable and be more than a little scary. Remember, those seemingly out-of-control behaviors are the reason that child is alive. These little people learned at far too early an age to do whatever they had to do to protect themselves.

The Gabriel's Angels staff works closely with the agencies' staff, because they are really the experts. If our therapy teams see or hear something that is unusually bothersome, they are instructed to speak to agency staff about it. At least one staff person from the agency is present for every therapy visit.

After a new therapy team has undergone initial orientation and has the perfect placement, one of our volunteer coordinators shadows them on their first two or three visits with the children. This is really a hands-on training experience, because knowing we have a great dog and a great person doesn't necessarily mean that the volunteer innately understands how to engage the children with their animal. The first goal is to establish a relationship between the team and the children. Unless and until we have established trust, we can't teach the core behaviors that intervene in the cycle of violence.

A little boy named Chance had lived at the Crisis Nursery for quite some time. He was an adorable blond guy with eyeglasses that were about half-an-inch thick. When Gabriel and I first met Chance, he looked at Gabriel and said, "Bad dog!" He then tried to hit Gabriel on his side. I quickly pulled Gabriel away from him, thinking, *My dog's not a bad dog!*

I soon learned that Chance's only experience with dogs had been with mean ones. In homes where domestic violence occurs, quite often the dog is also on the receiving end of the violence. And like the kids, these dogs' survival instinct can cause them to become mean. The dog Chance lived with wasn't a nice dog because it was getting beaten, too. This little boy's only experience of dogs was that they were mean. Over time, Chance began to understand that not all dogs were bad, including Gabriel. In fact, Gabriel was just there to love him. It was quite lovely to watch the relationship between the two of them develop.

* * *

Recently I attended a networking meeting where we were asked to tell the group one true thing and one false thing about ourselves. Then each person in the group guessed which statement was true. When my turn came, I said, "I jumped out of an airplane with a parachute!" and "When I was five years old, I was attacked by our family's St. Bernard." Knowing my love of animals and my sense of adventure, everyone immediately responded, "You jumped out of an airplane!"

Were they were surprised when my response was, "I've never seen any reason to jump out of a perfectly good airplane. Why would I do that?"

I told them it was true that I really was attacked by my St. Bernard when I was five. I had been watching *The Honeymooners* on TV and went out to the kitchen to get a mint Girl Scout Cookie. I got the cookie and then bent down to hug the sleeping dog. I scared him, and he came after me and bit me in the face. My dad held him back, and I went running to my room crying, dropping the cookie on my way. I've never felt the same about those Thin Mint cookies.

Innately, I always knew that incident was my fault. The dog was sleeping, and I woke him up and scared him, so he bit me.

What is interesting to me is that the situation did not instill a fear of dogs in me. I could have taken the attitude of, "That dog bit me, and I'm a victim of his viciousness." I turned out to be such a dog girl and to truly love animals as much as I do, but that incident could have shut me down forever. Although it was an important event in my life, I never gave it much thought until that networking meeting when someone in the group asked, "Do you realize how amazing that is? You were bitten in the face by a dog, so you have every reason to not like animals because of that. And yet you started an organization that utilizes dogs to help children. Classic Pam Gaber," they said.

Why was my response so different from Chance's? I'd had one violent encounter with an otherwise loving dog. For little Chance and so many other children like him, the violence is an everyday occurrence, and their pets simply don't know how to be loving.

* * *

Our volunteer coordinators are in the trenches with our therapy teams. "Our volunteers come from all walks of life," our East Valley coordinator explains. "Some have never worked with kids, so this is all new to them, and it can be awkward or challenging. I go with them on their first two visits. We help the volunteer introduce their dog to the children, telling them where the dog is from. We also discuss boundaries with the children, and how to treat an animal. We demonstrate the best way to approach a new dog."

After their first two visits, the volunteers come back to our office to receive training on how to use the activity kits we provide for each of our teams. Because our process is so intensive up front, our therapy teams are trained in the full range of behaviors they can expect to experience with abused, abandoned, and neglected children. For the most part, it will be hugs and kisses, but the reality is that we need to prepare them for all situations.

* * *

Debbie Coons is a former teacher who volunteers with her two bloodhounds. She works with junior high and high school kids and loves seeing the change that takes place in them once they become familiar with her dogs and learn to trust her. "I told the coordinator, 'Put me where you need me,'" Debbie says, noting that our volunteer coordinators "do a very good job at matching the volunteer and their dog with the right facility."

Debbie sees what every therapy team sees: some kids take longer than others to warm up to her. "Generally, the less trauma they've experienced, the shorter a time it takes for them to come around. It can be as few as two or three visits, or it can take as long as two to three months," Debbie says. "Eventually, though, the kids get to know the dogs very well. My dogs are littermates, but the kids can tell them apart just by looking at them."

While Debbie felt her dogs would be a good fit for Gabriel's Angels, she was still a bit surprised by how well they adapted to the work. "They just seemed to know which children to go visit. They would pick and choose, and the teachers would comment on how it was significant that they chose that child on this particular day." Debbie's bloodhounds resemble Gabriel, in that they are rowdy and rambunctious at home, but quiet, calm, and reserved when they're wearing their therapy vests and working. "I believe they really know what they're doing — that they're providing a comfort and a service," Debbie adds.

Debbie's most profound experience as a volunteer followed a gang shooting. One kid was killed just outside the school. "As we visited over the next weeks and months, the teens would get down on the floor to hug and nuzzle the dog. They wouldn't talk in counseling, but they would talk to me and my dog."

* * *

The ongoing management of our therapy teams is an essential aspect of our program. Because our teams do the core of their work through visits at the agencies, we don't see them all that often. Yet it's important to nurture our relationships with our volunteers and let them know we are always available to support them any way we can. After helping the kids, one of our biggest goals is making sure our volunteers have a great experience. We hold an annual volunteer recognition event and schedule quarterly workshops with our teams. We also host various events throughout the year to promote volunteer retention.

* * *

We have implemented agency agreements with all of the agencies we service. Recently, a woman contacted a local domestic violence shelter, looking for information about volunteering there with her dog. The shelter told her, "We have an agency agreement with Gabriel's Angels. We only accept therapy dogs that come through them."

Many agencies would agree with Marsha Porter's assessment that we are critical to their success; they know that pet therapy works, but they have neither the time nor the staff to manage their own pet therapy programs internally. It's a great testament to all the work we have put into developing our pet therapy program that these agencies have been willing to make Gabriel's Angels their gold standard for volunteer teams.

Gabriel's Angels now serves about sixty percent of Arizona children who would benefit from pet therapy. We currently partner with one hundred and two agencies and have one hundred and fifty therapy teams in Arizona. Teams either visit weekly or biweekly, depending on the volunteers' schedules. In the case of biweekly visits, a second team fills the gaps in the alternating weeks. Our goal is for every child we serve to visit weekly with a therapy team. Sometimes the agency has both an after-school program and a pre-school program. In those cases, we support both programs.

Three years ago there was a change in the state's child welfare system. In the past, kids would be placed in a crisis nursery and stay there for one day to forty-five days or more. A successful public-awareness campaign was launched in Arizona to inform our citizens about the need for foster parents. The premise was that children do better in foster care than they do in an institutional residential shelter. What troubled me, though, was wondering how Gabriel's Angels would be able to reach these children. Insurance requirements prevent us from visiting private family homes, due to what could be an unsafe situation if other dogs were in residence. I wondered how we could continue to touch these children. I went to the people I know in the child welfare arena and asked, "Where are they going?"

"They're going to foster homes and attending Head Start programs." Bingo! We had the opportunity to visit children there. I asked our program department to contact the director of the Head Start programs serving Arizona. We are now partnering with Head Start, and are working hard to meet the need. One program has fifty-two classrooms. At our current rate of placing five teams a month, it's going to take a year to fill the need. We're doing the best we can, and if we receive more funds for capacity-building, we'll jump on it.

* * *

Not every person is cut out to volunteer with abused kids. Over the years, I've heard a number of people say, "I could never work in the child welfare arena. I could just never work with children who've been abused. It would make me feel so bad, and I would cry. I would be heartbroken, and I just couldn't do it." Here is the most important lesson I've learned: I am no different than anyone else. My heart isn't any colder or harder than anybody else's, but this is not about me. If I can help kids, then I had better get over my "Poor me, I could never do that" story.

My heart has been broken by the situations I have seen, but I get stronger every time I see a therapy dog break through and reach a child. The people who say they can't do it — in my opinion, they're making it about themselves. If you can help a child, or if your dog can help a child, "I just couldn't do it" really isn't a very good excuse. This mission has got to be bigger than you. The whole point is that we're trying to help the children in our community. I feel as bad as anybody else when I see a child who's been hurt or scarred, but I'm doing something about it.

* * *

Mary Jo Dhein is a new Gabriel's Angels volunteer; she and her cockapoo, Goldee, started working with us in the fall of 2010. As an educator, Mary Jo has had lots of experience working with children, and she's seen, first-hand, the horrible and lasting effects of domestic abuse. Her dual passions to help kids and work to end domestic violence made Gabriel's Angels a natural choice for her. Mary Jo volunteers at the Sojourner Center in Phoenix during their Mommy and Me activities on Friday nights. "I visit with the children and the moms," she says. "I found out that the moms really enjoy the visits. I think that's because it's a chance to see their kids smile."

Asked why she volunteers, Mary Jo puts it simply: "I believe very strongly in volunteering. This combines my love for kids and animals. What could be better?"

Goldee also loves volunteering. "We'll pull into the parking lot, and she tries to get out of the car, because she knows we're there," Mary Jo explains. "It was Friday of New Year's Eve weekend, and we wound up cutting our visit very short. On the drive home, Goldee just laid down with her head on my lap. She wanted more time with her kids."

CHAPTER FIFTEEN

Gabriel — Film and TV Star

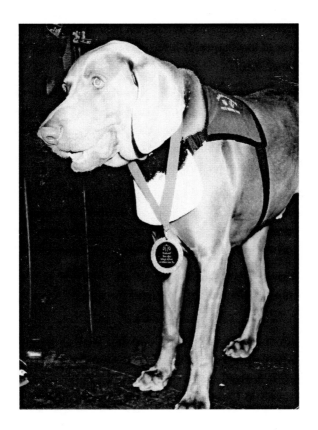

Years ago, Gabriel was featured in an international documentary called *Humanimal, the Animal Mind*. Its main premise was to highlight the fact that animal intelligence is far superior than once was believed. According to the website:

> For centuries, the animal world and the human world have been carefully kept separate. Humans once considered themselves to be at the

summit of intelligence and sensitivity, denying "beasts" all possibility of intelligence and emotions. Yet, as researchers and scientists make one discovery after another, they gradually prove that the border between the two worlds is not quite as impenetrable as once thought.

Animals can learn, memorize, imitate, dream; they have language, intuition, can adapt their behavior to a given situation, sometimes use tools, develop codes and systems of social organization. All these abilities require the solicitation of elaborate mental functions and the mobilization of intelligence. It is therefore no longer absurd to speak of the "animal mind."

In examining the anatomical and physiological properties of animals' brains, behavioral observations, research protocols and experiments undertaken by certain scientists, this series raises the foremost questions about animal intelligence and attempt to answer them within the confines of current knowledge.

How can this intelligence be measured? What is the reference for comparison? On which criteria? How can intelligence demonstrate itself? What does animal intelligence teach us about ourselves, human beings, and our world? And how do humans use this animal intelligence?

The documentary series profiled six different species: the pig, the wolf, the dolphin, the rat, the dog, and the ape.

* * *

The phone at the office rang one day, and on the other end was a man with a British accent: "Hello, is this Pam Gaber?"

"Yes, this is she."

"My name is Quincy Russell, and I am calling from Versailles, France."

"Hello, Quincy Russell," I answered, totally thinking someone was playing a joke on me, as this guy clearly did not have a French accent. "What might I do for you?"

"We are filming a documentary about animal intelligence. I work for a company called Mona Lisa Productions, and I have been on your website…"

I interrupted him to ask, "So, what time is it there in Versailles,

Quincy?" It was the quickest way I could think of to get a feel for wheth-er this guy was legitimate.

He answered, "It's about 3 p.m.," which was exactly what it should have been. *Maybe this guy is for real*, I thought. He went on to say that he wanted to profile Gabriel's work as a therapy dog with children in crisis in his film. He noted Gabriel's innate intelligence in reaching the children who needed his help the most. *Wow!! We're going to be in a docu-mentary!*

* * *

Quincy and his wife, Marie, flew to Phoenix to film Gabriel and his work with the children. They arrived on Memorial Day weekend 2003 to begin the project. Quincy wanted to open with a parade of therapy dogs entering the Crisis Nursery. I called all of our teams and asked them to come out. Every team showed up for the filming, and it truly felt like we had hit the big time. That was Day One. We spent the next two days film-ing Gabriel with the kids. Quincy got him interacting with a small group of children as they gently brushed his teeth and listened to his heartbeat. In allowing them to care for him in this way, Gabe brought out compas-sion and empathy in the kids — ideal for what the film sought to depict. I was so proud of Gabe!

Quincy was a rather adventurous soul, which is probably a good trait for a documentary filmmaker. His next idea was to film Gabriel in my car with his head out the window, as we drove into the nursery parking lot. If he could be adventurous, so could I. We gave it a go.

With Marie at the wheel of their rented minivan and Quincy hang-ing out the side door, we drove side-by-side down a relatively busy street in Phoenix. Quincy held his very expensive camera propped in place on his shoulder with one hand, while his other hand gripped a han-dle inside the vehicle so he — and the very expensive camera — wouldn't end up on the pavement. To this very day, I'm surprised we didn't get arrested for driving down the street like that.

Prior to Quincy and Marie pulling up beside my SUV, Gabriel has his head out the window, enjoying the summer air as he always did. So here came daredevil Quincy, hanging out of the rental van with the camera, trying to capture Gabriel on film with his head out the window. As soon as Gabriel saw the van with this crazy person hanging out the side door, he ducked back inside the car. Every time the van fell behind us, out popped Gabriel's head. As soon as the van pulled up beside us, Gabe would pull his head back in, like a turtle going into its shell.

We went on like this for quite some time, driving up and down the street. People who were walking stopped and pointed, "They're filming a movie!" But every time that camera got close to him, Gabe would pull head back in. Unfortunately, even after all that effort, we never got the shot.

Other than that, Gabriel did a great job. He was always good on camera. But then, at the end of the second day of filming, Quincy said, "OK. I'm ready to talk with you now." The last thing we had to pull off was an interview between Quincy and me. As you may recall, I was not nearly as comfortable as Gabe on film, but I was going to give it my best shot.

I sat on a nice comfy couch, and Gabe was to sit on the floor beside me. At one point, while Quincy asked me a question, Gabriel pawed at me, as if to interrupt. I looked over and said, "Almost done Gabe. Just a few more minutes." I swear he rolled his eyes at me. Then during one of my answers, he pawed me again, a little harder this time. I looked at Gabe and he looked at me, then the soft couch, then at Quincy. He looked at the couch and then at me and then at Quincy.

Quincy asked, "What does he want?"

"He wants to lay on the couch. Is that okay with you?"

"Sure!" he said. So lickety split, Gabe was up on the couch, laid down, and fell asleep in my lap. I continued my interview in peace, and Gabriel got a much deserved nap.

* * *

Gabe's star continued to rise. In 2005, I received a phone call from another young man with a British accent. He was from *Roadtrip Nation* and was quite excited that he was going to be in the States. "You know," he said in his British accent, *"Roadtrip Nation* — it's a bus. A bus that travels around the country. My name is Matt."

All I said was, "Okay, Matt."

"And we talk to interesting people."

Again, "Okay."

"And we want to talk to you."

"Okay." Wait a minute. "What??"

"And we want to come to your house."

That made me sit up straight. I tend to be a very open, trusting person but the idea of having some strange kids come to my house? No thanks. So I said, "I don't know. I'm really going to need more information, because I've never heard of *Roadtrip Nation*." Matt told me it was a PBS show.

"Well, it's not that I don't trust you, but I'll need to do some investigating of my own," I responded. I asked him if he could call me back in a day or so.

I did some research via the PBS website and found out that *Roadtrip Nation* is a TV show featuring college students who are trying to find their way in life, but not through traditional channels. They are not abandoning college, but they're interested in meeting people who have found their passion or niche and are leading exceptionally fulfilling lives. These students had searched the Internet for interesting folks, and somehow they came across Gabriel's Angels — and me. They learned how I had decided to leave the for-profit sector and serendipitously, with the help of a puppy, entered the nonprofit sector and created a life of meaning.

Matt called me back, as promised, and I told him, "I learned a lot about *Roadtrip Nation* and would be delighted to speak to you and your travel mates."

When I first found out they were coming, I went back and researched which other participants had agreed to these interviews. People from all walks of life: entrepreneurs, artists, musicians, writers, athletes, designers. Even some movie stars. For the original show in 2001, they interviewed Howard Schultz, the founder of Starbucks. One of the most prominent Arizonans they'd profiled was Jerry Colangelo, then owner of the Phoenix Suns and the Arizona Diamondbacks. And now they were coming to see me!? Once I realized how big this show was, it really made me nervous. Why would they choose me? I mean, they had the guy who started Starbucks! But this was Matt's project, and I was the one he wanted to talk with. He was young, but he wanted to find his passion. His burning question was: "How do you know when you have found your 'Why?' in life?"

Matt told me, "We're starting off in New York and will be winding up in San Francisco, via all the other places we're stopping. So we're looking to be in Arizona in about three weeks. I will call you about three days in advance, so you can plan for our visit." We decided the best thing would be to meet at the Gabriel's Angels office.

The crew kept in touch during their travels, and Matt called to tell me they would be in Phoenix the following Sunday in the late afternoon. A monsoon storm was predicted for that day. A summer monsoon is a dust storm followed by high winds and rain. Shortly after I arrived at my office with Gabriel and Mike, this HUGE lime green bus pulled into the parking lot. I looked up at the ominous gray sky; without a doubt, the monsoon was coming our way. We made it into the office just as the rain began to pelt.

Mike had driven Gabriel separately so that he could take him home after the interview. It was very hot and humid outside, but the air conditioning in the office kicked in. The boys met Gabriel and showered him with hugs and pats. The plan was for the boys to conduct a sit-down interview with me about how I had discovered my passion for roughly thirty minutes. There were two Matts on the team, but the one who called me took the lead because he was the one who had a deep interest in the nonprofit sector. As we sat for the interview around the boardroom table, we could hear the thunder and rain roaring outside. "Sorry, guys," I said. "Welcome to the Arizona monsoon."

"That's OK," they reassured me.

The lights began to flicker as the rain continued to pour down. I prayed that the power would stay on, as it had become dark as night outside, and without electricity there would be no air conditioning. BOOM! We heard a loud clap of thunder, and then the lights went out for good. My first reaction was, *Oh no*. But what came out of my mouth was, "I'm almost sure we paid our electric bill!" It was just the right comedic relief, and everyone busted out laughing.

In the dark, I found my way to the big front window and opened the blinds. The camera man — who was doubling as their chaperone — promised me that it was enough light to shoot by, adding that this incident would make for a very interesting interview. Without the air conditioning, the office quickly started to heat up, and Gabriel began breathing heavily. We did a test and discovered that we could hear his panting on the audio. Since it was now very dark and no one could see him anyway, Mike took Gabe home. He had performed his duty: he'd done the meeting and greeting.

We were all wondering, *Now what should we do?* We had only gotten through, at most, fifteen minutes of the interview.

I was thinking, *Wait! I didn't even get to the good stuff yet, and now we have to stop? This is my one chance to talk with these kids!*

So we all took our chairs over to the picture window where, with no electricity, they continued to film. One-half of my interview, which aired on national television, took place in the dark. "This is the most natural thing. This is how it happened, and we're going to roll with it. We're just going to keep going," said the cameraman. I sensed that they all shared the attitude of accepting whatever circumstances came their way and making the best of them. Probably a good philosophy for a *Roadtrip Nation* crew.

We continued with the interview until it became so dark that all you could see were strange shadowy movements. However, the audio was clear throughout. Once we'd wrapped up, the rain stopped and I walked out to their bus with them. They had a tradition that each person they interviewed wrote a message on the ceiling of the bus. I looked around and saw messages from all over the country. What a neat thing!

What I wrote on the bus was, "Shame on he who did nothing because he thought he could only do a little." I wanted them to leave with that thought. The whole experience was really interesting, and humbling, because before they arrived, I had been thinking, *What if I don't have enough of a story for these kids?* After the interview, I knew I'd successfully explained what Matt most wanted to hear: that I hadn't taken a traditional route to find my passion.

CHAPTER SIXTEEN

Helping Hands

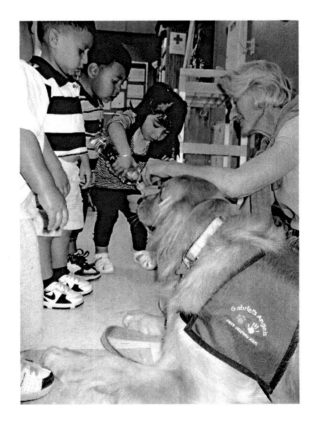

When Gabriel's Angels was first getting started, if you didn't have a dog to partner with, you were out of luck when it came to volunteering with the kids. Office help? Sure. But we had no other opportunities to work in the field with the children. After hearing from a number of people who were not dog owners but who really wanted to work with the kids, I wanted to develop a way for non-dog owners to volunteer at the grass roots level of our organization. As a result, we created the

Helping Hand position, where volunteers work as assistants to existing therapy teams.

Gabriel's and my Helping Hand was Linda; Gabriel knew her as Auntie Linda. For the last five years of Gabe's career, she came with us on every visit. She monitored little hands that roamed around in our activity kit. She helped the kids line up to feed Gabriel carrots and green beans. Upon Gabriel taking a carrot from a child, Linda would say, "Perfect!!" The children loved Auntie Linda. I don't know that I could have done a visit without her. I became quite dependent on her being there, and Gabriel did, too.

As Linda drove into the parking, Gabriel would begin to whimper inside my SUV. As soon as I opened the back door, he would fly out and run to her. And I'll tell you, nothing made her feel better than that. Even though he knew his job was interacting with the kids, the attachment he formed to Linda was incredible. Her heart was indeed broken when Gabriel passed away. We have learned that there's this undeniable bond between the Helping Hands and the dogs they work with. I've seen it at work for quite some time now, and it still amazes me.

We pair Helping Hands with the teams similarly to the way we place a team. People might say, "I've worked with teenagers before. I want to work with teens." In my opinion, our volunteer coordinators do an excellent job at pairing Helping Hands with teams because they get to know all the volunteers so well. Every year, the Helping Hand program continues to grow, because people want to give, whether or not they have a dog in their family.

* * *

As Linda tells it, "I had just gotten to a point in my life where I was going through a rough patch, and I decided I was so blessed that I needed to be giving back." Coincidentally, right around that time, Linda and I met at a local women's business group known as WISK (Women I Should Know).

At the time, Linda had a dog that was very sickly and she was unable to join Gabriel's Angels as a therapy team. I sugggested, "Well, what about a Helping Hand?" Linda asked me what that involved, and I urged her to attend an orientation meeting. After that, I invited her to work with Gabe and me.

"You always thanked me for coming, but I always went away with more than I felt like I was giving," Linda says. "And of course, Gabe always sensed when I wasn't having a good day. He'd hang close to me, even though we had all these kids on the playground." I would ask Linda what was wrong — and she'd tell me, "It's between Gabe and me."

Linda seemed to have a different bond with Gabriel than I did. After Gabe retired, she didn't get to see him much, but she really missed him. She asked me to let her know the next time he would be with me at the office so she could come by for a visit. "I knew I was going to see Gabe, so I went and bought a toy," Linda says, "and it just looked like a big, gray chenille worm. I got there and said to him, 'This is for you Gabe.'"

Gabe got that toy out of the bag, went and lay down on his bed in my office, and just proceeded to rip the thing to shreds. I tried to stop him, and Linda said, "No. Don't you know what's happening?" She believed he was venting all the frustration he was feeling from the medicine and the poking and prodding and chemo, everything he had just been through. He literally devastated the toy — we had stuffing all over the room. When I tried to pick it up, Gabriel came over and kind of booted me out of the way, like "Just leave it alone." I think Linda was right — you could feel the frustration pouring out of him.

I always marveled that he got so attached to Linda, because she saw him twice a month for an hour. They had such a terrific bond. Linda was heartbroken after Gabe passed. She says she never went back to say goodbye to the children at Crisis Nursery "because I wasn't the focal point — I was just the helper, part of Miss Linda and Miss Pam. It was Gabe who was the star." I asked her if she wanted me to get her involved with another team, and she just said, "Pam, I can't. It's too hard." Eventually, though, she called me and said, "I have a surprise for you."

"What's that?" I asked.

"Hook me up with another team!" I was so glad to hear that, but I completely understood when she said, "I just needed time, because I missed Gabe so much."

* * *

Our therapy visits are very Montessori in nature, hands on and age appropriate. For example if a child is not sharing, we see an opportunity to remind them to share the leash with the other children. There is really no such a thing as a typical therapy visit, as they vary based on the children's needs. One activity is not more important than another.

Sometimes the children would say, "We want to brush Gabriel's teeth." Gabriel wasn't a fan of it, but he tolerated it. I'd have to stand behind him because otherwise, he'd keep backing up until we moved across the whole playground. But he was gracious about letting them brush his teeth, almost as if he felt like it was what they needed to do. They'd help each other put the toothpaste on the toothbrush, and more often than not, Gabriel would lick it off as fast as they could put it on!

Other days, they just wanted to hug him. An all-time favorite was when Gabriel would go down the slide with the children. He had such fun!

CHAPTER SEVENTEEN

Learning to "Ask" for the Kids

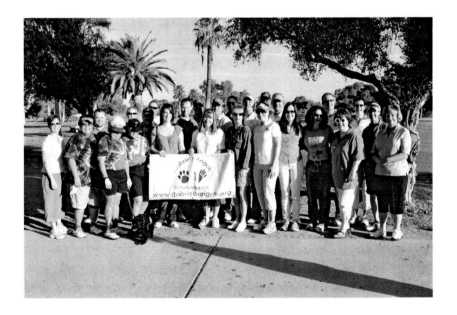

Though running a nonprofit has similarities to operating a for-profit business, there are some distinct differences. A nonprofit organization like Gabriel's Angels does not exist to provide profits to its owner or shareholders. We are a mission-driven organization that exists to provide pet therapy to children in crisis. The profit we do make is held in reserves in preparation for an economic downturn, or it's put back into the organization to improve our services. I love the concept that our profit does not go to staff or anyone else. It is used to make us better at what we do, therefore enabling us to leave the world a better place.

However, we incur expenses just like any for-profit entity, and we, too, must pay for the tools we need to run our nonprofit business. When I first started Gabriel's Angels, the phone company would have the nerve to send me a phone bill, and I would think, *But we're a nonprofit!* Guess what — I still had to pay the phone bill, pay the Internet bill, buy ink cartridges and office supplies, pay for postage, etc.

Mike and I made the decision that I would not take a salary, and we were able to do that for the first eight years. I was blessed, in that my corporate job had paid well and I had never had the time — or desire, really — to spend any money. Sure, there was always a part of me that thought, *I could have a set of Louis Vuitton luggage if I wanted it,* but I never felt the need to be seen with a brand. I'm not knocking people's preference to purchase exclusive brands, but it's just never been me. I always felt that running Gabriel's Angels was such a blessing. Being a part of enabling therapy dogs to heal children was all the pay I ever needed.

As we grew to twenty teams, and then to thirty teams, I was trying to deal with media calls, figure out how to raise money, and train and place therapy teams. I just couldn't keep doing it all, so we hired a part-time volunteer coordinator. We made the leap from just hard expenses to an employee, who obviously needed to be paid. We applied for a grant to help pay our employee, and we got it! Mike and I were still putting money in, and we'd get donations in dribbles here and there, but this truly was a shoestring operation.

And then, of course, the golf tournament came in, which was huge. Soon thereafter, we held our first 100-hole golf marathon, which involves hitting one hundred holes of golf in one day to raise money for the kids. Between those two events, we brought in about fifty thousand dollars that year. It felt so good to have the community show they believed in what we were doing.

It's always been my belief that the more money a nonprofit like Gabriel's Angels brings in, the more a community should rally around to support it, because it means the organization keeps getting better. This is another huge distinction from the corporate sector, where profits are distributed to upper-level staff and shareholders. I begrudge no corporation for making profit generation its focus. I just want those corporations with heavy profits and people with expendable income to invest back into the community. And Gabriel's Angels is a great place to start!

Our Animals and Children Together Learning Project activity kits are all funded by grants specifically written for that purpose. All the items that bring the children into close contact with the therapy dogs, such as brushes, stethoscopes, water bowls, doggie toothbrushes and toothpaste, are furnished to our teams at no cost to them. We do ask our teams to pay for their therapy dog registration, Gabriel's Angels t-shirt, and Gabriel's Angels therapy vest for their dog.

The process of becoming a therapy team — from that first phone inquiry to receiving training and being placed at a facility — is very intensive and time-consuming. And if we were going to continue operating, I was going to need funding to keep the lights on, train volunteers, grow the organization, and pay staff — which is probably the most important piece, because my staff drives this agency. We have now reached the size that on an annual basis, we schedule an external financial audit. The expenses to run Gabriel's Angels are legitimate; they are neither excessive nor glamorous.

Unfortunately, the mentality in certain donor circles seems to be, "We don't want to fund people; we want to fund programs." This perspective seems to miss the point that when funders are only willing to put money toward programs, you often wind up with a great program that languishes inside a poorly run organization. Lots of organizations have great programs, but if they don't have an equally fantastic commitment to the operations that run the programs, their whole existence can be jeopardized.

My measure of excellence is how well I meet my mission — how many children we help and the quality of pet therapy they receive. Business planning sets our strategic direction, and we know that running the organization well requires great people working at reasonable salaries. I can't imagine trying to approximate a well-oiled machine on some beat-up card tables and an old copy of Windows 98.

We've been very successful with our grant-writing program. Today, we bring in about forty-six percent of our total income through grants. I attribute our success to recognizing early on that most grantors want to fund specific items in a program. We build our grant program around how much money we need to fund a therapy team, because that's tangible to a funder: it's a person and their dog. Every $2,500 we bring into the organization goes directly to recruiting, training, placing, and managing a therapy team for one year.

I had to develop a reason for people to give. Paying the power bill to keep the lights on, or buying pencils and file folders isn't very sexy for a donor, so the secret was letting the grantor know that if we received a $10,000 grant, they would be enabling us to place four therapy teams for a year. I figured out a way to have donors help with enough of the operational costs to allow me to go out and raise the rest of the funds. It was a fairly ingenious way of doing it, but I didn't know how else to make it work. We don't need stuff; we need help with teams. To this day, it continues to be a successful program.

Donor funding helps with part of our operations, but we rely on our fundraising events to pay for the rest of our operational costs. These donations are not restricted in any way; these donors are saying, "Let's support the organization any way we can." When we receive these monies, we are honest about where they go. Because I had never really been involved with charitable work prior to founding Gabriel's Angels, I didn't enter this sector with preconceived ideas, like, "We're just a non-profit, so we shouldn't have new computers," or the thought that we should have any less than what we require to do our jobs. I've always been amazed when I encounter a bright business person who says to me, "Your teams are all-volunteer, so why do you need funding?" *Are you kidding me?!*

My standard answer is to appeal to their business mind that understands a balance sheet and a Profit-and-Loss statement. While we do deliver our service via volunteers, they must be professionally trained and managed, especially due to the fact that they are working with their therapy dogs among children. Core behaviors are instilled in the children with intent and repetition. This is never taken lightly at Gabriel's Angels.

* * *

One of our earliest fundraising events was our annual Doggie Beach Party in the Desert, back in May 2001. I have to be honest; it wasn't my idea. I swiped it from *Animal Planet*. One day I saw a show about a dog bakery in Seattle where they had a doggie beach party. I thought, *Hey, we could do that here; we don't have any water, but we can have a doggie beach party in the desert.* So the event became part of our marketing and fundraising strategy.

We held the first one on the blacktop parking lot behind a dog bakery. It was a hot day in the desert, so we had little wading pools scattered around. I have pictures of Gabriel in a Speedo and sunglasses! We drew about 60 people and their dogs. All the dogs played in the pools and loved it. We had a bathing suit contest and best body contest. Over the years, the event started to gain something of a following, to the point where we'd have maybe five hundred people attend.

One year, rain was forecast for the event day, so we purchased a rain insurance policy. It did rain on the day of our event, too — but it didn't rain enough. It rained just enough to cause all the to people stay home! In order for the coverage to take effect, we had to have 0.2 inches of rain at the airport. According to the official measurement, we had 0.14 inches. So we lost $1,400 on the insurance policy and most of our profit.

The annual Doggie Beach Party in the Desert was incredibly successful at getting us media attention. Three weeks before the event, I'd feel like I was on tour. I did every radio show, went on TV, sat for newspaper interviews — and what we learned through the years is that we never made very much money on that event, even though it was a lot of work. What it did do for us, however, was get us on the map with the local media. Now, we can make one call and get a story when we need to; we no longer have to jump through hoops. It was cute, fun event, but we've outgrown it. It was important to recognize the event for what it did for us, and then move on without a sentimental attachment to our very first formal fundraising effort.

Our second fundraising event was scheduled for two weeks after 9/11. We were as traumatized as the rest of America after the tragedies, but from a practical standpoint, we didn't know what to do. Should we cancel the event, or go ahead with it? It was to be an elegant affair with a band, appetizers, and a silent auction. We decided to hold it as scheduled and, well, it was not very successful. People were staying close to home, and it was just the luck of bad timing.

GABRIEL'S ANGELS

Our first attempts at fundraising events were not rousing successes, but we kept pressing on.

* * *

We shifted to a different strategy: a large fundraising luncheon. The first few years, we held the event at the Stone House Pavilion at the Phoenix Zoo, a lovely room that overlooks the zoo grounds and seats three hundred people. Gabriel was permitted to come to the zoo to represent the Gabriel's Angels' therapy dogs. Interestingly, this zoo, full of animals, had restrictions on dogs, even service dogs, because of fears that the dogs would bring in diseases that their exotic animals might contract. My thought was, *Well, I'm just as nervous that the monkeys or giraffes could give something to Gabriel!* The zoo does allow service dogs, but those visitors must be accompanied by a guide the entire time.

Upon arrival, Gabriel and I went to the front entrance to let them know we were there. At this time, he had finished his chemo treatments for his first bout with cancer, but he'd been prescribed some Prednisone, which gave him a ravenous appetite. So here he was, my perfectly behaved therapy dog, the founding dog, and that day he jumped up and ate a chocolate cookie out of the hand of one of our donors. Then he promptly walked around the corner and barked hello at a service dog he encountered. All of this, while I was speaking to our three hundred assembled guests. I suddenly heard "Cling, clang, clank," and "Woof!" Sometimes these things just happen when pets — or kids — are involved.

* * *

To be successful in running a nonprofit organization, you must succeed at asking people to support you. This idea of asking can haunt even the most confident people. The thing is, Americans give habitually to organizations and causes they care about. They expect to be asked. In 2007, Americans donated $306 billion to charity. This means that two-thirds of all households contributed funds to nonprofit institutions. Charitable giving has withstood the test of time in our country. As all levels of government decrease funding and challenging economic conditions persist, the case for nonprofits strengthens.

Learning all of this was a process for me. When I first started, it was difficult for me to ask people for money. Somehow, even though I knew my mission was serving the children, it still felt like I was asking for myself. I had to shift my perspective, and I now ask for money for the little people we serve. I ask donors to make an investment in our community, for our future, and for the future of our children. Thinking about the unconditional love our pet therapy teams bring, and the way they build empathy in the children we serve, I have no problem asking for help. The message I convey is that it's a privilege to be a funder for an agency that is helping children exit the cycle of violence. Usually the only reason someone hasn't given to charity is because no one asked them.

* * *

Wayne Anderson, DVM, is one of our major donors. Our fundraising consultant, Mary, introduced me to him because she thought he would be a good addition to our steering committee. She was right! Wayne started off by sponsoring a therapy team — and soon sponsored several more. "To recognize me," Wayne says, "they made the hike all the way out to my office and presented me with a plaque to say thank you. I thought that was really neat. So now I have several plaques on my wall from the therapy teams I've sponsored."

One of Wayne's fondest memories is going with Gabe, his wife, and me to visit to the Crisis Nursery before Gabriel started slowing down. "It was very exciting to see Gabe, the therapy dog, in action. The most memorable part for me was just the giggling of the kids. Some of them would sort of back off, but then they'd start at the other end — they'd start at the tail and work forward, giggling the whole time."

Wayne sees his role at Gabriel's Angels as one of connector. "My role, I think, is to expand the sphere of Gabriel's Angels. All of these kinds of organizations need money to do their work — but the heavy lifting is done by the volunteers. You don't get money if you don't have volunteers. The thing about Gabriel's Angels is that it serves more than one hundred organizations that work with at-risk kids. So when you give to Gabriel's Angels, you give to one hundred programs all at one time."

* * *

At Gabriel's Angels, we have trained all of our board members on the "Culture of Philanthropy" so they can get comfortable with asking on their own, as well as accompanying me on major donor visits. I always take a board member with me on visits to potential major donors. The thing is, I have a vested interest in getting that donation, but the board member is someone who is strictly a volunteer — they didn't start the organization — but they donate their time, talent, and expertise to sit on our board and they fully support us. That matters to potential funders. Each board member can now answer the question of why they support Gabriel's Angels and articulate it with enthusiasm and passion.

* * *

Our board members come from all segments of our community. Some are older, some younger. Some own businesses, while others are retired. All share a couple common traits: an unbreakable, loving bond with their pets and the desire to help Gabriel's Angels continue to make a difference in the lives of the little people in Arizona.

Robert Burghart, incoming chair for the Gabriel's Angels board, got involved with Gabriel's Angels after finishing his MBA. "During school, I really enjoyed the conversations I had about how to change things, and I missed that when I finished. So I figured the best way to continue those conversations and actually see the words in action was to start doing some sort of philanthropic service." Fortunately for Gabriel's Angels, Robert chose us as the place he wanted to make a difference.

"Originally I thought I would just make a donation and learn a bit about the organization. Once I saw Gabriel's Angels and the passion everyone involved has for it, I thought it would be very interesting to be part of a small organization that I could watch grow, and see what I could do to have an impact." Since Robert has been involved with us, our budget has grown to twice what it was when he started, and we've probably doubled our staff.

"We had a bit of a downfall due to the recession," explains Robert, "but we had some forethought. We saw what was coming and discussed what was likely to happen from a standpoint of the effect on charitable giving. We knew that we needed to be cognizant of our spending. So I think that although we took a hit, we had two things going for us. One is that we were watching for the shift and we were prepared for it. Two is that we had been in such a strong growth mode over the previous few years that we were able to sustain our programs and services.

"When you really boil it all down, one of the most important things we do is plan ahead, because we don't ever want to go somewhere and initiate therapy teams just to pull them back later due to budget issues. We always make sure that we're on track to remain consistent in our services. I credit our board and executive staff for making sure that when we make decisions, we look at them from a couple of angles so that we know they're sustainable."

Like many of our board members and other executive staff, Robert has been on visits with therapy teams. We feel it's essential that all of our personnel — from the office staff to the board to the steering committee — understand from the inside exactly what Gabriel's Angels is all about, so they can know exactly why they are involved.

"When I think of my interaction with Gabriel's Angels and my tipping point with the organization," Robert says, "I credit it to Gabriel. I went on a visit with Gabriel to the Crisis Nursery and I got to see Gabriel interact with the kids. It was like the adults were invisible, at least initially. The kids were there to see Gabe. But watching Gabe, it was as though he knew what he was doing. He introduced us as the adults, and brought us into the interaction. He would either pull us closer to the kids, or pull the kids closer to us. He worked with the kids, but made sure we were right there, involved in what was happening.

"What Gabe was very good at, in my opinion, was being the conduit between the child and the adult. There were many times Gabe would help us talk to the child or help the child open up to us. And when the child was doing something he wasn't supposed to be doing, Gabriel would just look at us. He knew his place. He wasn't there to discipline anybody; he had a great way of bridging the communication between the child and us. He just seemed to innately know what he was doing. He was conscious that he was helping us in our work with the children."

CHAPTER EIGHTEEN

First Bout with Cancer

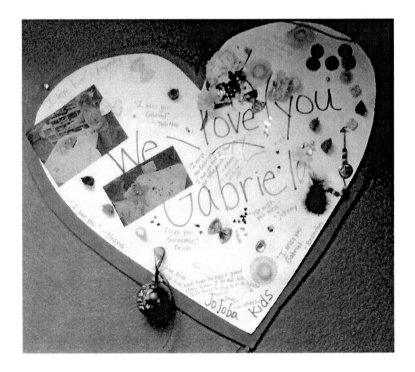

When Gabriel was about two years old, I noticed a small, fatty tumor right above his rear leg and abdominal area where this little fold of skin hung down. I could feel each side of this little pea-sized bump. I checked it periodically, and it stayed the same size for years, but one day I thought it seemed a teeny bit bigger.

Gabriel was then five, and while we were at the vet for a routine teeth-cleaning, I told Dr. Rice, "I think it's growing a bit." It felt like it was maybe the size of a pea-and-a-half. I said to Dr. Rice, "You know, I feel it every day. I look at it every day. I don't even see Gabe anymore — I only see the bump. I want it out." Dr. Rice agreed, so he cleaned Gabe's teeth and removed the mass. He sent the specimen off to the lab as a precaution, because I wanted confirmation that it really was only a fatty tumor. This was on a Tuesday.

The following Friday morning, the Dr. Rice's female vet partner, Dr. Fitzpatrick, called. I answered, "Hello?"

She asked, "Are you sitting down?"

"What is it?" I asked, immediately panicked.

"I am sorry to tell you that Gabriel's tumor was malignant." It was a Stage III mast cell tumor.

"Are you sure?"

Dr. Fitzpatrick said, "I wish it wasn't true, but you've got to get him to an oncologist. We recommend Dr. Betsy Hershey. We didn't get clean lines so he will need a second surgery. But let's not get the cart before the horse." (The term "clean lines" refers to surgical cuts that correspond to the membrane surrounding the tissues.)

I took a big breath and said, "OK, give me the number." I hung up in shock. I immediately got back on the phone to the oncologist, and her receptionist answered. I told her my dilemma and wanted to arrange to bring Gabriel in ASAP, like *right now*.

In a calm voice, the receptionist said, "Dr. Hershey can see you at the end of next week."

"I don't even know how I'm going to get through the weekend, so I really need to see Dr. Hershey before that."

"I'm sorry, but she doesn't have open appointments."

"Well, I'll tell you what. This dog is the founding dog of Gabriel's Angels." I figured I'd try name-dropping. If it worked, it would be worth it.

She said, "Oh, I've heard of Gabriel's Angels."

"This is Gabriel," I said, "and I'm pleading. I'm begging you. I have to come there on Monday. I will come and sit in the office on Monday morning. I will be quiet. And if Dr. Hershey has a cancellation, she'll be able to see Gabriel." It was cool outside, I reasoned, so Gabriel could wait in the car. "But I will sit there until she can see us. I promise I won't cause any trouble, but I will come in on Monday morning."

The gal said, "I don't have anything, but just a moment. I'll be right back." She came back on the line and asked, "Would three thirty Monday afternoon be okay?"

"Three thirty on Monday would be fine." I exhaled and thanked her sincerely. Then I hung up the phone and began to cry. I petted Gabriel's big head, and he looked at me, as if wondering why I was so sad. There he was, now being the consummate therapy dog for me. That amazed me. He didn't know that he was the cause of my angst. He thought I was sick or upset, and he kept trying to relieve my obvious sadness.

I started to worry that he might be spending too much of his energy comforting me, and not enough on getting well. I realized I had to pull myself together and somehow let him know I was fine so that he could focus on his healing. I made the decision to get over my worry so Gabriel didn't have to keep taking care of me.

By this time, Dean Rice, our vet, had become a close personal friend. He gently informed me that a mast cell tumor is not unlike breast cancer. It can be easy to catch and treat, or it can be really invasive. Gabriel required chemo and radiation, and it took a while for him to respond.

* * *

Unwittingly, I became a part of a new community, a community of people who take their dogs in for chemo or radiation. You sit in the room and you talk, because you share the common bond of trying to save your beloved pet. I remember there was one Great Dane — a Harlequin — that had an osteosarcoma. He'd had his front leg amputated, but he didn't know it. He'd come bounding out of chemo, so happy to see his owner. His owner was a big guy, and each time he would brace himself as this huge dog came running toward him.

I bonded with the other owners whose pets were in treatment. The schedules do not vary much from week to week, so we would see each other often. Gabriel received intravenous chemo one week, and would then have the next week off, except for a blood draw. The week after that would be oral chemo, and then a week off, except for the blood test. That was our schedule for more than five months.

The week off between treatments was critical, because cancer drugs can be very toxic. If Gabriel's white blood count was in the normal range, he could receive chemotherapy the next week. It was really quite a sophisticated process. One time Gabriel's white count was below five hundred, so he was unable to receive chemo that next week. The time between treatments was occasionally extended because Gabe sometimes needed ten days in between treatments to recover.

Through this experience, I learned how animals simply accept their circumstances, unlike humans who complain when we have a hangnail. To witness the way animals just deal with whatever life brings their way was such a privilege.

* * *

About midway through the cancer treatments, Gabriel developed the canine version of Bell's palsy: the left side of his face was just hanging there, and from what we could tell, he had minimal feeling. I freaked out when I noticed his left eye drooping and that he had no blinking reflex. I immediately took him to the vet and asked, "What's wrong?" They were not sure. We would touch his face, and his eye wouldn't blink. Nothing.

Though they were never able to diagnose precisely what was wrong, the vet's office told me to monitor Gabe's condition and gave me drops to put in his eye so it wouldn't dry out. Poor dog couldn't get a break.

A few weeks later, the right side of Gabriel's face also began to sag. Not as badly as the left side, but it was noticeable. My vet immediately sent me to a veterinary neurologist in town. I know it wasn't my normally optimistic way of thinking, but my only thought was, *He's going to have a brain tumor.* The neurologist told me that if the preliminary tests indicated further testing, she would recommend a CAT scan. First, though, she just did several simple tests. She took Gabriel outside to watch him walk around so she could check his balance. His balance was fine. She performed a various other tests and concluded that he had the bilateral canine version of Bell's palsy. The neuro vet reassured me that while there was no known treatment for the condition, dogs usually recover over time.

Dr. Hershey recommended we give acupuncture a go to alleviate the Bell's palsy. At this point, pretty much anything was worth a try. So while Gabriel was undergoing his chemo, she would perform acupuncture. She inserted the needles: a couple in his head, a couple in his lips, and a couple in his feet. "I think this will help the big gray dog," she commented.

One day, I went to pick Gabe up, and Dr. Hershey said, teasing me, "He tried to bite me today."

"What!?"

Again she said, "Gabriel tried to bite me."

"What were you doing at the time, sticking needles in his head?"

She smiled and said, "Yes, as a matter of fact, I was."

"Well, fair enough!" Poor Gabe was getting a little testy with all he was going through.

The next time he was scheduled for acupuncture, Dr. Hershey said, "Let's try having you stay with him to see if he handles it better." We had him sit on a bench instead of an exam table, and she began to insert the needles while I held him in my arms and patted his head. His right muzzle began to curl up, ever so slightly, though the left side remained flat.

"See?" she said. "He's looks like he's ready to bite me!" The only reason we knew he was irritated was because his right side had a little movement.

"You know what, Doc? He's using his words."

And his words were, "I don't want you doing that." He never did bite her, but we always laughed about that. We decided to stop the acupuncture because all it seemed to be accomplishing was stressing him out. Eventually the right side came back, but the left side of his face was always a bit flaccid.

* * *

The high doses of Prednisone caused Gabriel to drink a lot of water, and thus urinate quite frequently. He also lost some weight during all of this. Generally, animals undergoing chemotherapy don't lose their hair or get nauseated. My best guess to describe how he was feeling was achy and puny.

Due to the frequent urination, I took him with me almost everywhere I went. Every thirty minutes or so, he had to go out. It was three days after Gabe's oral chemo treatment, and Mike brought him to a Gabriel's Angels board meeting because we didn't want to leave him alone.

I noticed that Gabe seemed to have this lavender aura around him. It was so strange. His tongue was lavender, his gums were lavender, and he just didn't look right at all. His eyes were huge. I was concerned and took him to the vet the next day. That's when we found that his white count was below five hundred. The vet put him on antibiotics, because he virtually had no immune system function. After that, we didn't take him anywhere for a long time.

* * *

It was amazing during this time to find how the Universe just has a way of taking care of things. I felt like a full-time soccer mom driving my kid from place to place. In spite of putting in many hours at Gabriel's Angles, I somehow found the time to take him to chemo every week and for blood work in between. I'd wait for him, take him back home, and then go to work. I was also making sure the teenage boys were still seeing Noah, my other therapy dog. I guess you just find a way to make it all happen.

One monumental lesson I learned through all of this was that I hadn't really understood how deep Gabriel's bond was with the children of Crisis Nursery. I always saw it, appreciated it, and loved it. I knew he was a rock star in their eyes, but when he was sick and couldn't visit his kids, they were terrified. "Where's Gabriel? Where's Gabriel? Where's Gabriel?"

The staff did not hide the fact that Gabriel was sick from the children. They told the kids, "Gabriel's sick, so he can't come visit you right now." The children made him a big card. The adults wrote down what each child said. I've never forgotten Michael's comment: "I love him and I miss him and hope he has a good day. When I grow up, I'm going to buy him a house and a bone."

Others simply said, "We love you."

"We miss you, Gabriel. We hope you come back. Adrian."

"We don't want him to be sick."

The staff asked me to come to the nursery to talk to the kids about Gabriel and explain to them how he was doing. Initially I said, "I can't. I can't. I'm too upset."

They gently prodded me, "You need to come. The children need to understand that Gabriel did not abandon them, that he is sick and you are okay." Put that way, how could I say no? That was when they presented me with the big heart card the kids had made. It made me cry, and I remember being embarrassed about that. The staff told me, "It's okay to cry, because they need to know how much you love Gabriel."

The words, kind thoughts, and get well wishes meant a lot coming from those kids. It really did. I also learned that, yes, the relationship was deeper than I'd ever realized. It was also eye-opening to me that this organization was flourishing and continuing to heal children, even though Gabriel wasn't in the spotlight.

CHAPTER NINETEEN

"Gabriel Gets His Wings"

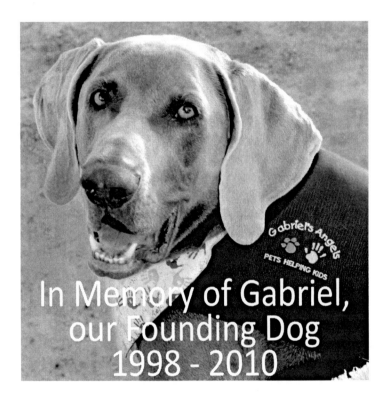

In Memory of Gabriel,
our Founding Dog
1998 - 2010

It was August 2009, and Gabriel had just returned home from his visit with the kids. We were in the backyard, and I noticed something on his left front leg that looked like a little bump. Since he'd already had cancer several years earlier, fear swept through my body. I panicked and touched the bump; it felt kind of hard. I worried, so I called my veterinarian that afternoon and got Gabriel in to see him the next day.

GABRIEL'S ANGELS

Dr. Rice had sold his practice and was now working at the Phoenix Zoo. Dr. Pullen looked at Gabe's leg and felt the mass. To play it safe, we agreed to remove it and scheduled the surgery for the next day.

Gabriel was in surgery for two-and-a-half hours. It seemed like a long time for such a small mass. It turned out to be tumor — we don't know where it originated — that had traveled like a worm throughout Gabriel's leg. It was approximately four inches long! While growing, if it hit a tendon or a bone, it would stop and simply go around till it found more tissue to consume. The tumor took the path of least resistance, so it wound up above his wrist area, finally protruding out where I could see it. Apparently, what I thought was a small bump that had been there a day or two had probably been growing for six months or more.

This cancer was different from his first bout, which is why I believe Gabriel had the cancer gene. The first one was a mast cell tumor. This one was a hemangiopericytoma — a fibrous, nasty, gnarly mess that was impossible to remove completely.

We gave Gabriel some time to recover from the surgery and several days later went back to see Dr. Hershey. I didn't have to threaten to sit in the waiting room this time; she knew us well by now and saw Gabriel immediately. Though I was glad to see her, I would have preferred to do it under just about any other circumstances.

She gently petted Gabriel and told me that we had four choices. One was to do nothing. *Yeah, right.* Two was to amputate his leg all the way up to the shoulder. The third choice was radiation under anesthesia every day, Monday through Friday, for a month. He'd have weekends off. The last option was chemotherapy injected into the place in Gabe's leg where the tumor had been, twice a week for the first two weeks and then once a week for a month.

In my opinion, none of those choices was a good one, so I had to rank them. Doing nothing was not an option. To amputate the leg of an eleven-and-a-half-year-old dog seemed harsh, due to his age. If he had been a young dog, I might have felt differently. Five days a week of radiation under anesthesia also was a poor option, due to Gabriel's age. The intralesional chemo seemed like the best of four bad choices.

Mike and I talked it over, and I explained that the intralesional chemo meant putting the chemotherapy drug directly into the area where the tumor was. Very little would be absorbed systemically, so we decided that was the best of all the choices. We arranged for Gabriel to begin the chemo after his sutures were removed. The trips to see Dr. Hershey brought back memories and tears. Here I was, again trying to save Gabriel's life.

We began with twice-weekly visits for the chemo treatments. I found solace at my office, which was nearby, so I would go there until he was ready to come home. Somehow, the brightly colored walls of the Gabriel's Angels offices and my amazing staff brought me peace. Besides, it doesn't really work for the boss to be a crying mess.

Gabriel was lightly sedated, as the chemo was being injected directly into his leg. Because the injection site was near the wrist area, his skin didn't have a lot of pliability. As a result, Dr. Hershey could only inject so much of the drug because the skin began to pull tight. She was never able to deliver all the chemo that was recommended. We kept at it, though, hoping for the best. Gabriel was a trooper, and all seemed to be going well.

Sure enough, we made it through the treatment. I was cautiously optimistic as his wrist remained swollen until the chemo was absorbed. The swelling finally subsided completely soon after his last treatment. Gabriel made a visit to see his kids at the Crisis Nursery in January 2010. He was so excited to get in the car, but once we got there, he ran out of steam. His mojo was off and he obviously lacked enthusiasm. The children were so happy to see him. They hugged him and kissed his head. But that was the day I realized that it was time to retire my Gabriel.

The dog who had inspired a revolution, leading hundreds of therapy dogs to begin healing children in crisis, was done doing what he was born to do. But it was the right decision, and I knew it. I wanted him to have a happy, stress-free rest of his life.

A few weeks later, his wrist was swollen again. I took him back to the veterinary surgeon, who told me he could do surgery again, but putting Gabriel through that stress was not appealing. We went back to Dr. Hershey, who said, "You can try to keep doing surgery, but at this point, I don't know what else we can do. I'm not sure how long he's got, but I think he should go home and have a great life. He could be fine for a year or two."

Mike and I were devastated, but we knew we had done all we could for Gabriel. He was acting pretty much the same, so we banked on "a year or two." Thoughts swirled through my mind: *Should we have amputated his leg? Should we have done radiation?* It's easy to second-guess yourself, but as I look back now, I still think we did the right thing by choosing the intralesional chemo.

About a week later, he started coughing. If Gabriel had been a cat, I would have thought he had a hairball. All of a sudden he would hack, and I'd see a little bit of blood on the floor. Sadly, I made another appointment to see Dr. Hershey. While we were in the waiting room, he started to gag. No blood, but at least the staff heard the sound he'd been making at home. When I took Gabe back to the exam room, unbeknownst to me, the technician had already told Dr. Hershey, "He was choking in the waiting room."

Dr. Hershey said to me, "Please have a seat in the waiting room. I want to take a quick chest x-ray." She took Gabriel to the back, and I went out to the waiting room. I was scared and didn't know what to think. I thought he might have pneumonia or an upper respiratory infection. In about twenty minutes, Dr. Hershey called me back into the exam room, and I heard soft music filling the air. My heart froze, as there had never been music playing before, and I thought, *This is not going to be good.*

The music simultaneously scared me and irritated me. I found it anything but soothing, so I hit the off button. I didn't want to listen to that. Dr. Hershey returned with Gabriel and said, "I'm so sorry, but the cancer has spread to his lungs." She had really just been trying to comfort me with the music. We looked at the radiographs of his lungs. Where normal lung tissue is black, Gabe's was white. I could see the lumps and the bumps. Again she said, "I'm so sorry. There's really nothing we can do now. Pam, you gave it your all." This was toward the end of February.

Then she said, "I want to take an impression of his paw."

"Why?" I asked. "What for?"

She was insistent, "We're going to take an impression." Only weeks earlier, she had said "a year or two," so I thought he still had lots of time, but things had changed and she knew better now. She took his paw impressions and kept them, and I didn't hear much about it after that.

* * *

As a canine oncologist, Dr. Hershey noted how different the two cancers were. "Gabriel's first tumor was a mast cell tumor, which is a very common skin and subcutaneous cancer in dogs. It's rather rare in people, but it is common in dogs. What was ironic in Gabe's case was that the mast cell cancer can often be very unpredictable. We see a lot of dogs that develop metastatic disease or spread from the mast cell, but he survived that particular cancer.

"The second cancer was actually a connective tissue malignancy," she continued, "the biggest challenge of which is trying to control them locally, where they grow. Gabe's tumor was down on his leg, where it's hard to treat because you can't take it out cleanly, so we were left with trying to do some adjunctive therapy. He had his surgery, but we couldn't get the whole tumor. Given his age and the fact that he was still working to some degree, we decided against radiation and wound up treating the remaining cancer with intralesional chemo — injecting the chemo right at the surgery site. He actually tolerated it much better than we thought he might. But the tumor grew back very rapidly, even between chemo treatments. Now, normally, that type of tumor has a very low potential to spread, but in Gabe's case, that's exactly what happened."

* * *

In March 2010, Gabriel woke up in an absolute panic in his crate. He was panting heavily. I let him out, and he slept on our bed. Occasionally he would have bouts of panting, and then he would be OK. When he did sleep on our bed, he spread way out on his side, probably because he was uncomfortable. He took up the whole bed.

One night there was no room for me, so I slipped out to catch some sleep in the guest room. Later Mike called to me, "Pam! It's Gabriel — there's something wrong!" Gabriel was hyperventilating to the point where half of the entire bed was just soaked with saliva. He was panting so hard that he couldn't catch his breath. I sat for two hours with his head on my lap and just petted him, and he finally calmed down and went to sleep.

GABRIEL'S ANGELS

In the ensuing months, there were good days and there were bad days. There were days when we thought he was going to make it, and there were days when he could barely breathe. He was still eating fine, though, and even carried around his beloved blue ball. Whatever Gabriel wanted, he got; we were at his beck and call.

Mike and I hiked the mountain near our neighborhood about two weeks before Gabriel passed away. The desert has a special vibe for us. While hiking, I could tell he was crying but didn't want me to know. When we got all the way to the top, Mike said, "We're going to have to put Gabriel to sleep soon, aren't we?"

It was my turn to be strong for Mike. I said, "You know, it's not today, but we have to grasp this, because this is the reality. This is the reality." He nodded his head and looked out at the horizon. He didn't speak all the way down.

* * *

Several months prior, I had called Gabriel's first vet, Dr. Dean Rice, and I asked him to meet with me. Over coffee, I told him we'd found out that the cancer had spread. I asked him, when the time came, if he would come to our home to relieve Gabriel of his suffering. I couldn't stand the thought of taking Gabe to a vet hospital for that. For one thing, Gabriel was already too freaked out over hospitals, as he had spent so much time there lately. Also, it just didn't feel right. Dean said he would come to our house whenever I needed him. I was so relieved.

And at that point — to lighten the mood just a bit — I said, "Gosh, Dean, I feel like I just made my son's funeral arrangements." It was surreal.

I would occasionally call Dean at all hours, sometimes panicked because Gabriel was having a bad day. He always reassured me, "He's fine for now, Pam. Trust me, Gabe will let you know when it's time."

It was Sunday, May 16, 2010, when I made the final call. "I really know it's time. Can you come over tomorrow?"

He said, "I can come over at 6 p.m."

Monday was the saddest day, but we knew we were doing the right thing. What would life be like without my big gray dog? Oh, how I was going to miss him. I spent all morning with Gabriel, telling him it was going to be okay and that I would be fine without him.

* * *

During Gabriel's second bout with cancer, I had located an animal communicator with excellent references. It had never occurred to me to utilize such a person, but a friend recommended I try, if only for my own sanity. Starting shortly after the second cancer diagnosis, I would speak to Sage weekly, asking, "How's he doing? How is he feeling?" She said he was somewhat unaware of what was going on, but she kept focusing on what she perceived as pain in his left shoulder.

I kept telling her, "Sage, the tumor is in his left wrist area, not his shoulder." She didn't know the cause, just that he had discomfort in his left shoulder area.

Sage also recommended that I do more than merely talk to my dogs. "Converse with them," she advised. "Try to really listen to them, and see if you can pick up what they are feeling. What you should do is tell Gabriel that it's okay. Tell him it's okay. Tell him you love him, and you understand, because he will be more at peace if you talk to him rather than at him."

All these years, and I had never realized that I talked *at* my dogs, "Oh, you're a good boy," but I never truly conversed *with* my dogs. I do now.

Sage told me that one of Gabe's worries was about who was going to be in charge of the pack after he was gone. Sage got a message from him, as the patriarch of the house, "Don't let Jack be in charge."

She told me, "I'm getting communication from Gabe that he doesn't want Jack to be in charge after he's gone."

Well, that made perfect sense, because Jack had no skills to be the pack leader. Jack lives in the moment without a care in the world. In charge? I don't think so. But when she accessed Noah, Noah told her that he didn't want the job either. So Gabe was worried — who was it going to be? The cat? Orzo's nice enough, but he's not exactly large and in charge. It was really interesting, because through all of that, I really learned how to communicate with my animals.

I would arrange to talk with Sage about Gabriel while I was at work. But one time she said, "At some point, you need to be with Gabriel while I talk to you." So I arranged to be home for our next session. I was sitting on the ottoman in our family room, and Gabriel was sleeping on his bed in front of the fireplace.

I called Sage and said, "OK, I'm home."

"Let me access him and see how he is doing." Suddenly, Gabriel jumped out of the bed and desperately tried to get into my lap. There was no way this huge dog would fit in my lap, and he almost knocked me on the floor with his effort to climb on top of me.

I was so startled, I said, "Whoah!"

Sage asked, "What's wrong?"

"Gabriel is trying to get in my lap. He is frantic."

She explained, "Well, as I accessed him, he freaked out. He wanted to know, 'What are you doing?' He got scared."

"Yes, but he's in my lap!" This episode made me such a believer, because even though our conversations had been reassuring, I was still a bit skeptical about this whole animal communicator thing. But this was surreal. He had never tried to get in my lap before. Yet the minute Sage got to him, he had a reaction. He calmed down once he realized it was Sage. Sometimes, too, when she connected with Noah or Jack, she told me they would ask, "What are you doing? What are you doing?"

There at the end, I was petting Gabriel and felt underneath his left shoulder. I noticed a lump, about the size of an egg. Ah, that was what Sage had been talking about. It was his lymph node that had been bothering him. Yet I had kept insisting, "No, that's not it. It's not his shoulder." I'd felt that Sage had the special gift of communicating with animals, but it was more of a belief than from experience. Now I was so glad I hadn't dismissed what she'd told me about Gabriel and my animals. There was that lymph node, what she'd been describing as pain in his left shoulder, right where she told me it was bothering him. I was shocked.

After speaking with Sage, I told Mike, "You need to spend the afternoon with Gabe, and you need to tell him it's okay. That'll be the best thing you ever do for him because, Mike, he's got to know. I mean, he's a therapy dog, so he's got to know we're going to be okay." Mike did that, and as hard as it was for him, it was as good for Mike as it was for Gabriel.

* * *

Precisely at six o'clock in the evening on Monday, May 17, the doorbell rang. I opened the door and Dean came in with his big doctor bag. It resembled a fishing tackle box. All his life, Gabriel had never been a fan of having people walk into the house. Workmen? He didn't like them. This was his house with his people, and no one else should enter.

Now, though, Gabriel was breathing very heavily; it was time, and I was so very sad. Gabriel saw Dean and spun with delight. He even wagged his tail. He was so happy. He had known Dean from years ago, but it had been a long time since they'd last seen each other. I don't know if it was scent memory, or if Gabriel thought, "Here's my angel, because I cannot do this anymore."

I think our timing on all of it was impeccable.

We got Gabriel into his bed in the kitchen, and we talked a little bit. Gabriel loved the kitchen, as he always wanted to be where the action was. I said to Dean, "I owe you my life, because the only alternative would have been taking him somewhere, and I just couldn't do that."

As he was talking to Gabriel, Dean gave him a sedative. Gabriel became really quiet, just looking at us. He was so sweet, and we were just petting him, telling him we loved him and that he was going to be okay. During that whole time, the euthanasia drug went in, and it was the most peaceful, beautiful passing. I mean that, because I felt such love. I felt such love and I felt certain that we had done the right thing for our dog. He just took a sigh, and suddenly he was asleep. Of course, we were all crying as I felt Gabriel walk across the Rainbow Bridge.

Gabriel passed away on Monday, May 17, 2010, at 6:29 p.m.

Jack and Noah were right outside the kitchen when Gabriel passed. We have glass French doors, so they could see everything. I made sure they saw it all. I didn't let them come in to smell the body, as I felt sure they understood what had happened. Amazingly, they also were fine with Dean being in the house, because normally when someone they don't know is in the house, they bark and make a fuss. With Dean, though, they seemed to know why he was there. I asked Dean to take Gabriel's body with him. He didn't take Gabriel — he took the body. We wrapped him in Mike's Green Bay Packers blanket.

GABRIEL'S ANGELS

Dean spoke recently about the difficult decision to put down a dog. "It's a tough decision," he explained. "It's a quality-of-life issue, which is a real subjective decision to make. But it's my job, as a veterinarian, to advocate for the animal, because they can't speak for themselves. I've had to do this a number of times in my career, and it bothers me every time. But then I realize that if I get used to it and it doesn't bother me, I should quit this work altogether."

Dean says that most people hope their dog will just die peacefully in its sleep, but that usually doesn't happen. "I think that's happened maybe a half-dozen times in my entire career, which is why it's up to us to intervene and not let the animal suffer. The animal will let you know, but the other half of the equation is that the human has to be ready to let go. If we've established the point, medically, that we can't do anything more for this animal, we need to be honest. And when I got there that night, Gabe was glad to see me. He knew, and I knew. It was time."

People sometimes ask if I have Gabe's ashes. I don't. I didn't want them, because his spirit was what made Gabriel. His body housed that incredible spirit, but in the end, his body betrayed him. I didn't want the ashes, because keeping the ashes would mean holding onto the cancer. I have no regrets at all about that. I don't need his ashes to feel his presence.

Back when I'd met with Dean, he asked me if I was going to want Gabriel cremated. At that time I said, "I don't know," because I had never lost a pet like Gabriel and I wasn't sure. I did wonder if I might regret not having the shrine. But I've never for one second regretted it. So when people will ask, "Do you have the ashes?" I simply say, "No. I feel him every day, and that is good enough for me." I just feel so much more spiritually connected to him this way.

* * *

From September 2009 until May 17, 2010, I continued to run Gabriel's Angels while trying desperately to save Gabriel. As if this was not emotionally and physically draining enough, things were about to get even more challenging. On April 15, 2010, I received a call from my dad that my mom was in the emergency room. Three days later, she was diagnosed with Stage IIIB cervical cancer and was told she needed treatment immediately.

Chemotherapy and radiation were the protocol, so we dove head first into that. *I can save her, too,* I thought. I now had my "once in a lifetime dog" in the late stages of lung cancer and a mother with late-stage cervical cancer. It was full throttle between my mom and Gabriel, yet I never missed a day of work.

Mom knew Gabriel wasn't well, but that was all she knew. It was late March when she said to me, "Pammy, when you have to do something with Gabe, and you have to put him to sleep, can I be there? I love him so much and I want to be there. Do you think that would be okay with Mike?"

"Of course you can be there," I told her, sensing how very important it was to her to hear that. Little did we know what lay ahead. Here she was, wanting nothing more than to comfort my pet, with no clue that right at that moment, she was dying, too. My mom loved Gabriel like a grandma loves her grandson. I caught her once closed inside the pantry with Gabriel, giving him doggie treats. She and I even gave him his first bath. They had such a special bond.

Mom was back in the hospital when Gabriel passed away, and I couldn't even tell her. She was so sick that I couldn't bear to give her any bad news. I had to meet with her chemo doctor the day after he was gone as if nothing had happened. Maybe I'm a better actress than I realize, because one said anything. As it turned out, we didn't tell her for a week. I needed to mourn Gabriel's passing, but I couldn't, because I had to be upbeat and ready for Mom, in order to help her through her own process.

Finally, when she was released, I had to tell her. "I don't want to upset you. I know that you're feeling good today, but you need to know that Gabriel passed away." She just started to cry, "Oh my Gabey." I never really had time to deal with my own feelings about him, but maybe everything does happen for a reason.

I took Mom a Gabriel's Therapy Dog Trading Card to put in her room when she went back into the hospital. She was so weak, and she knew the end was near, but she told me, "Pammy, I am going to see my Gabey."

"Yes, Momma, you are."

I take great comfort in knowing they are together. Whenever I see a cloud, I think of them. Someone once told me why God made clouds:

when the animals are done playing beyond the Rainbow Bridge, they circle three times and lay down on the clouds. I see clouds now and think, *Oh, Gabriel's sleeping there.* My mom passed away on July 25, 2010. To lose them so close together made me feel so much more a part of humanity.

Now I go into a restaurant, look around, and think, *Every one of these people has had something happen in their life. They have stories too.* Or, when I was visiting my mom in the oncology ward, I would sit with her and think, *I'm not the only one. We're not the only family. I'm not the only woman who lost the most absolutely amazing dog who ever lived. Nor whose mom is dying of cancer.* That's what I've taken from this whole horrific experience, that I feel human. I feel very empathetic toward people. It also changed my communication with my pets. I converse with my dogs now, not just talk at them.

* * *

I continued my talks with Sage, following Gabe's passing, always asking, "How is he? What's happening?"

"I won't know anything for a couple of days," she explained. "They just don't communicate immediately, but once he crosses over, I'll know. So I'll just keep accessing, and I'll let be in touch."

A few days later, she called me and said, "Gabriel has passed beautifully. I see him as kind of a trampoline dog. He's so happy and light. I see a little muse. He's a muse." I told her that every once in a while, I can feel this warmth, kind of like a stuffed animal, but with no stuffing, wrapped around me. He comes and he leans on me, and I talk to him. I'm so happy — and relieved — that he's happy. If I had to guess, he is heading up all activities over the Rainbow Bridge. Losing Gabriel took a part of me, too. Godspeed, Big Gray.

* * *

Now I realize that the whole idea of animal communication may be foreign or weird to some people. I suppose I wasn't really a true believer until my own experience. I asked Sage how she would explain telepathic communication to someone unfamiliar with the concept. Sage explains telepathic communication as "feeling across a distance. We all have that capacity to feel across a distance. It's similar to thinking me

about a friend or a family member, and then suddenly they call, and you say, 'Oh, my gosh. I was just thinking about you.'

"We all have the capacity to tune into that radio station belonging to another human being. Well, the animals have their own radio stations — they have their own level of communication. They communicate between one another very easily. And we all have the skills to communicate with the animals, too — it's just that we often shut it down at a young age. Kids connect really easily with animals because they are open to it. The skill I've fine-tuned over the years is to dial into that animal radio station and to hear what they are saying."

Sage explains that animals don't move their lips the way we humans do, but they do communicate. "Animals use a variety of ways to get their point across. I may hear words. I may see images. I might get physical sensations in my body — with Gabe, for example, I would get physical sensations in my body. The animals will communicate in whatever way they are able to get their point across. I just have to be open to listen to it."

At one point during our work together, Sage asked me if I was communicating with Gabriel about what was going on in his body. "Have you told him that he has cancer? And do you want to tell him?" She told me that we often assume that because we know that something is happening with the animals, that they know, too — but that some animals could really care less.

"It's we, the humans, who get really emotional about things. We have a diagnosis and a prognosis, while the animal's just chugging along, feeling okay. I listen more to what the animal says than to the prognosis. What I remember about Gabe was that he was okay moving on because he wasn't particularly tied to this life. I think he had something of a concept of death, but I had to explain it to him. He didn't have a whole lot of emotional attachment. He was such a Buddha dog. He was so willing to just let go, and it allowed his passing to be a little easier because he was ready and there wasn't anything missing for him."

While we were talking, Sage told me, "I just got a message from Gabe right now — all my hairs stood up. He's loving that this book is being written, and he's loving that we're having this conversation right now. He just randomly showed up, and he was like 'I love this.' He's really enjoying the attention. He wants everybody to know that he's having a lot of fun."

"What's he doing? Is he chasing a ball?" I had to know.

"I don't get that he's chasing a ball. What I get from him right now, in this moment, is a red-violet energy that's just zooming around. So I don't get a physical sensation of him chasing a ball — it's more just the energy of Gabe. It feels like he has such a sense of freedom."

* * *

After Gabe passed, the next adventure was waiting to see who would assume the alpha dog role in our home. The one thing we knew was that it would be decided by the dogs. Honestly, I don't think either of them wanted the job. Jack certainly didn't have the skill set — after all, another of his nicknames is Kramer, after the Seinfeld character. What's happened is that Noah has assumed the laid back alpha role. It's a subtle, "I'm in charge," attitude, which gives comfort to Jack. I am so thankful that it worked out the way that it did.

Since Gabriel's been gone, we've learned that Jack has separation anxiety. We didn't know that before, because somebody was always with him. If I took Gabriel to work, Noah was home. If I took Noah out, Gabriel was home. If I took Jack, he was with me. In three years, he was never alone in our home. Recently, Noah's had several veterinary appointments for an injured foot. With Gabriel no longer here, I had to leave Jack at home alone. He literally tried to escape. Trying to find us, perhaps? He even attempted to carve a doggie peephole into our mahogany front door. "Hey, maybe if I dig out a little hole in the door, I'll be able to see my people!"

One of our cats has his own room, and Jack crashed the gate down. He destroyed the plantation shutters trying to break out of the side bathroom. This is the most amazing, loving dog, but we've learned that he can't be left alone if we want to keep our house in order.

Recently I had a talk with Noah about his pending toe amputation because of osteomyelitis. I told him, "You know, buddy, they're going to take your toe. I hope you're OK with that."

He turned and looked at me, as if to say, "It's just a toe." I feel like now, when I really listen to Jack, Noah, and Orzo, they have something to say.

* * *

During all the drama — dealing with my mom, and Gabriel's passing — my staff said, "You owe it to the thousands of people connected
to our agency to let them know that Gabriel died." They meant everyone from the volunteers to the donors to the staffs at the agencies we'd
served.

"I'm not going to deny that it should be done," I said. "But I'm not
up to doing it. It can come from our office. I give you total permission,
and I know you'll do it properly." Our staff was mourning, too, and this
was going to give them a way to honor Gabe. They sent out an e-mail
to our 5,000 supporters to let them know about Gabriel, and it was the
right thing to do. We were shocked by the number of phone calls and e-
mails we received in response. Then the sympathy cards started coming
in. Most of them said, "I remember when I met Gabe." Or "I was here
when I met Gabe."

Then Connie Midley, a reporter from *The Arizona Republic*, called
and said, "Pam, our newsroom just found out about Gabriel." She
sounded very sweet, but a bit tentative, due to the sensitive nature of
her call. She continued, "My editor walked into our staff meeting, and
said, 'Gabriel of Gabriel's Angels died. I want to know if Pam can talk
about this.'"

I told her, "You know what, Connie? I can do it. I can talk about
Gabriel for Gabriel. I can do it for him." The article appeared on the
front page of the Living section, and the headline said, "Gabriel Gets
His Wings." It was the most beautifully written story I've ever read. Ga-
briel also made it into the *Business Journal*. Someone called me and said,
"That was the only dog I've ever seen eulogized in the *Business Journal*!"
But he was known about town, and he'd impacted everyone he met.

What I didn't realize along the way was how many people's lives
Gabriel had touched over the past ten years. It wasn't until all the cards,
phone calls, and e-mails started coming in that I truly learned the mag-
nitude of his impact. Gabriel's Twitter followers did a prayer circle for
him, and his Facebook fans mourned, as well.

* * *

In June 2010, I received a call from Dr. Hershey, asking me to come
by her office. By now I'd completely forgotten about them, but she gave

me the two impressions she had made of Gabriel's paws. She had decorated them with gems, his name, and also some angel charms. It was a bittersweet visit, as I had never been to her hospital without Gabriel. We both cried and reminisced about Gabe. I loved the creative thoughtfulness of her gesture. One of the pawprints sits on my desk where I see it every day. The other one is at home.

CHAPTER TWENTY

The Future of Gabriel's Angels

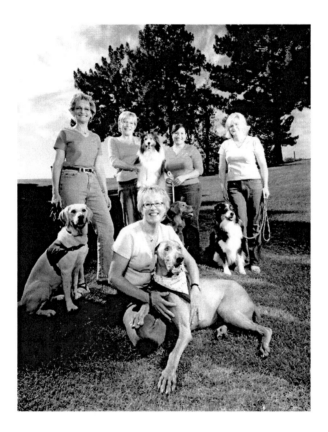

To be honest, I'm not entirely sure what the future of Gabriel's Angels will be.

We will, no doubt, continue serving the needs of the children of Arizona. We expanded into Southern Arizona and are now beginning to branch out to Northern Arizona, as well. We've received some funding from a foundation for that purpose. Also, we had a couple teams who moved up north, and they would like to continue working with kids under the auspices of Gabriel's Angels. Our research shows there are agencies we can serve in the northern part of the state.

Weekly, and sometimes more often than that, we hear from people who are interested in starting a Gabriel's Angels in their community. We'll get questions like, "Can we have Gabriel's Angels in Indiana?" Unfortunately, it's not quite that easy. The pet therapy side is easy — because we can always find great people with great dogs to volunteer. It's the funding that takes more effort and energy. Before opening in a new community, the most important thing is making sure that there is funding coming in to support the teams in these new areas of expansion.

I had a unique opportunity to start this organization, because I was able to quit my job and give it as much time as it took to nurture it. I'd been in training my whole corporate career to be able to do this, from both a business and a monetary standpoint. To develop a sustaining resource engine takes an extremely high level of commitment, business sense, and passion.

In many ways I felt as if I was in training my whole life to be able to run Gabriel's Angels and make it successful. That being said, you can never question where you are in a moment, because I know now that Corporate America was where I needed to be for those fifteen years. And when I wasn't supposed to be there anymore, I was supposed to be here. I would never have had the entrepreneurial spirit had I not already known how to run a business.

Would we like to see Gabriel's Angels go national? Yes. More than that, though, I'd like to shutter our doors forever because child abuse and neglect no longer occur. Unfortunately, that's not going to happen. And as long as there are children who remain in the cycle of violence, they will grow into parents who create new kids in crisis in need of our services.

* * *

Who is to say what the future holds for Gabriel's Angels? I do know one thing — that whatever happens, Mike Gaber will be at my side watching it unfold. Mike has been beside me, behind me, and with me through every step of this amazing journey. Without his support, it never would have happened. From behind the scenes, he has been so much a part of the unintentional success of Gabriel's Angels, from adopting that big, gray puppy to watching him become the dog who inspired a revolution. Mike still misses Gabe terribly — it's a loss I'm not sure he will ever get over. When I asked him to contribute a few thoughts for the book, he initially said no — it would be too hard. Eventually, though, he realized that it would be one of the best ways he could honor Gabriel's legacy:

> What was most special for me was watching the progress Pam made when she initially left the corporate world and started doing some human volunteer work with the Crisis Nursery, and then as we brought Gabriel into the household, and then the genesis of the whole project when she introduced him to the kids during that Christmas party. The propulsion that took off from there was astonishing, in how the organization grew.
>
> When you look at Gabriel, you see how he grew into his role. It was pretty powerful, because he went from a dog that was just having fun at home to, quite frankly, a dog with a professional canine career. He had a career that spanned his lifetime. Just to watch that and to see how seriously he took that job — it was truly impressive.
>
> Another thing I saw first-hand was how we were able to form the organization and really mold all the other therapy teams and their dogs after what Pam had created with Gabriel. Because when you look at the footprint of the organization, everything is tailored after what she and Gabriel started out with, progressed with, ultimately accomplished, and I would say, actually perfected. That formed the template for how Pam created the organization and how all the other volunteers and their dogs fit into it.
>
> It was really an intuitive thing that Pam did, but what made it work was that she had a very intuitive companion and partner in Gabriel. Here's the best way I can put it: Had our only dog at the time been Jack or Noah, neither of them would have had the capacity to engage and think it through like I truly believe Gabriel did. I don't know that the organization would have formed and moved forward. I don't think either of them could have done what Gabriel did to create the movement. They fit into the organization once we got it going, but they weren't the types of dogs that would have been able to put it in gear.

And I think that might be true of a lot of dogs.

You'd have to go through quite a few dogs to find the next one that had the capacity to work with Pam the way Gabriel did to achieve the success they did together. That's my biggest take on how it started, and how it took off. They were able to fine tune each other — she played off of him and he played off of her. I think that is critical to observe, because without it, I don't think this organization would have had any legs at all.

Now it's just a matter of perfecting the growth Pam and Gabe began.

Resources

GABE'S AND PAM'S MEDIA APPEARANCES

Humanimal, the Animal Mind
http://bit.ly/humanimal

Roadtrip Nation
http://bit.ly/RoadtripNation

Money magazine article
http://www.gabrielsangels.org/news/RealLifePamGaber.pdf

EXPERTS MENTIONED IN THE BOOK

Phil Arkow
Instructor, Animal-Assisted Therapy, Harcum College & Camden
County College; Consultant, ASPCA & Animals and Society Institute;
Chair, Animal Abuse and Family Violence Prevention Project, The
Latham Foundation; Coordinator, National Link Coalition; !deas —
Communications Solutions for the Nonprofit Sector.
www.animaltherapy.net

Sage Lewis
Certified life coach; Level 3 Certified Tellington TTouch® Practitioner;
animal communicator; shamanic practitioner; fun person.
www.dancingporcupine.com

HUMAN/ANIMAL WELFARE

Human Society of the United States
First Strike — The Violence Connection
http://bit.ly/humane-first-strike

GABRIEL'S ANGELS

GABRIEL'S ANGELS SOCIAL MEDIA CONTACTS

Facebook
Facebook.com/PamGaber
http://on.fb.me/facebook-ga (Gabriel's Angels)

Twitter
Twitter.com/GabrielsAngels
Twitter.com/TherapyDogGabe

LinkedIn
Linkedin.com/in/PamGaber

YouTube
YouTube.com/user/GabrielsAngels

THERAPY DOG REGISTRATION

Delta Society
www.DeltaSociety.org

Therapy Dogs Inc.
www.TherapyDogs.com

STARTING A GABRIEL'S ANGELS IN YOUR CITY

If you are interested in starting a branch of Gabriel's Angels in your city, here are the things you will need to do begin:

- Form a 10-member board of directors, with officers.
- Meet your state's requirement for registering an established 501(c)(3).
- Develop a two-year line item budget.
- Research agencies in your area that would benefit from and be receptive to working with a pet therapy program.
- Create a fundraising campaign to raise 18 to 24 months of funding.

Once you have these things in place, we'll be happy to talk with you about the next steps. Reach us at info@GabrielsAngels.org or 602.266.0875.

CHILDREN'S LIST OF REQUIREMENTS FOR TAKING CARE OF A DOG

from page 81

These are some of the actions the kids routinely put on their list when we teach them about all that is involved in taking care of a dog:

1. Feed him.
2. Give him water.
3. Brush him.
4. Give him a bath.
5. Pick up his poop.
6. Play with him.
7. Walk him.
8. Clip his nails.
9. Take him to the vet.
10. Check his ears.
11. Brush his teeth.
12. Rub his belly.
13. Give him treats.
14. Teach him to sit, stay, down, and come.
15. Teach him tricks.
16. Give him a safe place to sleep.
17. Put a jacket on him if he is cold.
18. Take him for a ride in the car.
19. Take him to the groomer.
20. LOVE HIM!!

GABRIEL'S ANGELS

PUBLISHING RESOURCES

Bill Greaves/Concept West
Graphic design/Book design/Website design/Photoshop illustration
BillGreaves.com
bill@billgreaves.com
480.595.5510

Laura Orsini/Write | Market | Design
Editorial, marketing, and design solutions for socially conscious
speakers, coaches, and authors.
WriteMarketDesign.com
Facebook.com/writemarketdesign
laura@writemarketdesign.com
602.518.5376

Author Bio

In 2000, Pam Gaber founded Gabriel's Angels, a 501(c)(3) nonprofit organization. She recognized the pressing and documented need in her community to enhance the lives of neglected and abused children through the application of pet therapy. The organization was named after Pam's young Weimaraner, Gabriel, who began his career by visiting the children residing at the Crisis Nursery in Phoenix. During these visits, Gabriel offered unconditional, nonjudgmental love, teaching the children empathy, compassion, and respect. By watching Gabriel help the children to trust again, Pam saw that something life-changing was happening for them and felt compelled to reach more children.

The triumph of Gabriel's Angels is manifested in Pam's leadership position as CEO and her daily involvement in the development, growth, and vision of the organization. Presently, Gabriel's Angels has 150 Pet Therapy Teams serving more than 100 agencies and reaching 13,000 Arizona children annually.

Pam serves as Treasurer on the Board of Directors for the Humane LINK; sits on the Executive Committee for the Children and Animals Together Diversion Program and the Program Committee for the Organization of Non-Profits; and is an Athena PowerLink Mentor. Her achievements include winning the 2008 Hon Kachina Volunteer Award; recognition by *Arizona Foothills* magazine as one of the Women Who Move the Valley; being named one of the 2010 Women in Business by the *Phoenix Business Journal*; and selection as a 2010 Phoenix Chamber Athena finalist. In 2011, she was chosen as the YWCA Woman of Excellence in the nonprofit sector and voted Most Influential Nonprofit Executive by *Arizona Foothills* magazine.

She resides in Phoenix with her husband, Mike, and their two dogs, Jack and Noah. All are kept in line by Orzo, the resident cat.

9 780615 445908